THE
HOME
SECURITY
HANDBOOK

THE HOME

HOME

SECURITY

HANDBOOK

Expert Advice for Keeping
Safe at Home (and Away)

LYNNE FINCH

Foreword by Mike Seeklander

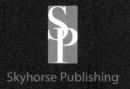

Skyhorse Publishing

Skyhorse Publishing books may be purchased in bulk at special discounts for sales promotion, corporate gifts, fund-raising, or educational purposes. Special editions can also be created to specifications. For details, contact the Special Sales Department, Skyhorse Publishing, 307 West 36th Street, 11th Floor, New York, NY 10018 or info@skyhorsepublishing.com.

Skyhorse® and Skyhorse Publishing® are registered trademarks of Skyhorse Publishing, Inc.®, a Delaware corporation.

www.skyhorsepublishing.com

10 9 8 7 6 5 4 3 2 1

Library of Congress Cataloging-in-Publication Data is available on file.

Cover design by Owen Corrigan

Print ISBN: 978-1-62873-742-4
Ebook ISBN: 978-1-62914-103-9

Printed in China

For Nichole, a loving friend who was wonderfully
supportive and will be missed.

CONTENTS

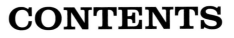

TABLE OF FIGURES

///

FOREWORD

If you knew me well you would realize I almost never read a book in detail. My time is too short. Instead, I look for material that is clearly written in a manner that I can act on. I look at chapter titles that contain information that I can directly, and immediately use. I am very picky about the material I spend time reading simply because I just don't have time to waste! My years of life have taught me that simple, easy-to-read, material is faster to act on, and action on any resource (outside of the world of fiction) is key!

The Home Security Handbook is the second title by Lynne Finch that I have read (the first being *Taking Your First Shot*, a must read for any shooter, especially females), and the one thing that stands out the most was the fact that I immediately began to scan for and find tidbits of information I could personally use, right then. My point may not become apparent until you realize that I am a former police officer, federal law enforcement instructor, author of two training books, one on defensive shooting and one on competitive shooting, numerous training DVDs of my own, and co-host of *The Best Defense* on The Outdoor Channel, a show that focuses almost entirely on armed, unarmed, and environmental safety. I am supposed to be an expert at this stuff, and I have access to a huge and very broad base of highly qualified people while filming the show.

And here I am, reading Lynne Finch's book and absorbing the material like it was new to me! Thinking "I can use some of these tips on *The Best Defense!*" The book reminds me about what I thought when I met Lynne—she is direct, polite, intensely analytical, and more importantly knows her stuff. After we met she sent me her first book. After getting *Taking Your First Shot*, I scanned the chapters and immediately began to jump to bits of information that I wanted to read. I was pleasantly surprised; this was a woman who got it right! It is an incredible rarity to find such knowledge and passion about shooting coming from a female outside of the competitive shooting world.

The book you are holding in your hands is filled with information. More importantly, that information is well researched, actionable, and may save your life. I always liked to tell my graduating students in my firearms classes at the Federal Air Marshal training center that the information we had given them was useless unless they took the responsibility to use it (continue to train) correctly. Read this book. Act on the information presented within it. Take responsibility for your own safety, because ultimately, the only real self-defense is individual. Please don't make the horrible assumption that it can only happen to someone else . . . it's a mistake you can't rewind when the wolf is at your door or worse yet, inside it!

—Mike Seeklander
Former US Marine, Law Enforcement Officer,
Federal Air Marshal, and Federal Firearms Instructor
Co-Host of Outdoor Chanel series *The Best Defense*
Owner of Shooting-Performance LLC

CHAPTER 1

INTRODUCTION

I've been studying personal defense and safety for many years and more recently began teaching and writing about unarmed and armed personal defense and shooting. This book focuses on ideas to make your home safer, whether you rent or own, as well as ways to keep yourself and your family safer at home and away. It doesn't matter if you are blocks away at the grocery store or hundreds of miles away on vacation, there are things you can do to help you be aware and to stay safe. We'll also look at the option of firearms for home defense, including selection, ammunition, and safe storage. For more information on learning to shoot and carrying a firearm outside the home look for my book *Taking the First Shot* from Skyhorse Publishing.

The world we live in has become very unpredictable, but there are things you can do to keep the odds in your favor. Being prepared is your best defense against something bad happening. Reading and implementing some of the strategies in this book is the first step on your path to making you, and your family, more secure.

Be safe.

—Lynne

CHAPTER 2

REINFORCING YOUR HOME

T here are many things you can do to make your home more secure. Most are low cost options that are not permanent and work equally well in a rental property or a home you own. Let's start with easy ideas to make a rental more secure—these can apply to any home.

EXTERIOR DOORS AND WINDOWS

Keys: First, and maybe most important, you don't know how many sets of keys may be out there, especially if you are in a large apartment complex. Ask that your unit be rekeyed (the lock changed so old keys don't fit anymore) *before* you move in. If you are there already, you can still ask that it be rekeyed. This is a relatively easy task for a locksmith and your landlord should understand that it is for your security. You may be asked to pay a nominal fee, but it is worth it for your safety!

Peep Hole: Does your front door have a peep hole, sometimes called a viewer? If it is a standard viewer you may not be able to see much, however, for a few dollars at most any hardware store you can buy a "wide-angle" viewer that affords you a much better view and it will usually fit in the same hole. Your existing viewer may also be very dirty and not give you a good view. A flat screwdriver is generally all it takes to undo the existing one. If you look at the viewer from the end there are usually notches; that is where the screwdriver goes to loosen the viewer and make it possible to switch it out for one that offers a better view.

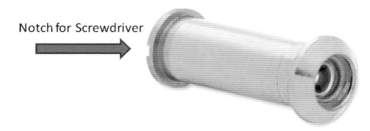

Figure 1 – Peep hole

Sliding Doors: These are particularly vulnerable if you don't have a brace for them. The simplest option is a dowel, about the size of a broom handle or slightly smaller, cut to fit in the track to block the door from sliding, which also makes it hard to jimmy and lift off the track.

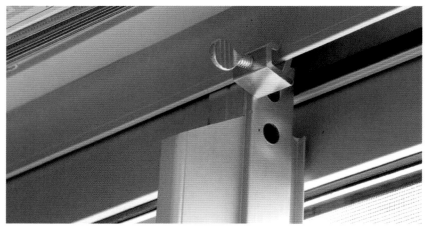

Figure 2 – Sliding door lock

You can use a telescoping security bar, similar to a tension bar curtain rod. And, there are screw mounted brackets that block the door and are hard to see from the outside that make it impossible to open the door (this can be great for keeping the little ones on the inside, too), but whatever block or locking device you use, make sure that any overnight guests are aware of them, and how to operate them, in case they need to exit the home in an emergency.

Main Door: For very little money you can install a brace that makes it much more difficult to force your door open, while allowing you to easily

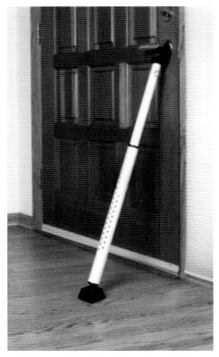

Figure 3 – Door brace

move the brace. There are braces that snug up under a doorknob and have a foot that resists sliding. Or, if your configuration is such that you have a wall or heavy piece of furniture, you can cut a board to size (or have the hardware store cut it for you), and brace the base of your door, making it more difficult to open.

Windows: You can secure the windows in a rental unit. You can get brackets very similar to that used for the sliding door shown in Figure 2, keyed or unkeyed, that slip on and prevent the window from being raised beyond the point where you have attached the lock. For older windows, a dowel can be inserted in the track or a nail can be hammered into the side to prevent it from raising beyond a limited range.

All of the suggestions above can be accomplished for under twenty-five dollars each, and do not leave any permanent changes to the property, except the nail which can be removed. In addition, you can take the door and window locks with you when you move.

Lighting making it look like someone is home!

There are lots of ways to make it look like you are home when you are not. Programmable timers have gotten much more sophisticated, and less expensive. You can get one that controls more than one light, you can even get them that program seven days independently with multiple on/off times. There is also an amazing little box that simulates a TV screen, changing color and intensity somewhat randomly. It is also programmable and you can put it in any room where the glow could be seen through a window and it will appear as if a TV is on. If you are really clever you can coordinate timers so that they go off on the main level and come on in the bedroom a minute later. These work not only if you are away for an extended period but if you work late and come home after dark allowing you to come home to a lit house.

If you own your property, there are things you can do, in addition to those depicted above, to reinforce your security. Do any of your exterior doors have glass panels or windows, other

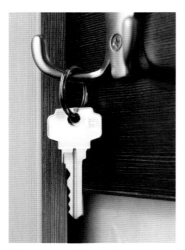

than the small decorative windows at the top? If so, consider double keyed deadbolts. These are locks that require a key to open, both from the inside and the outside. This prevents someone from breaking the glass and reaching in to unlock the door. I have French doors to my deck. They are double keyed and the key is attached to a decorative tassel and hung on a pretty hook around the corner and out of reach of the door. This does take discipline, you must always put the key back in the

Figure 4 – Spare key

same place so you can find it in an emergency.

There is a wonderful device called a Door Club that serves as a block at the base of the door, making it very difficult to force open but it does take a little more skill to install since you must drill into the floor. Once installed it rests against the base of the door until you step down on it to lock into place.

Door Hinges: Do you know that the average exterior door hinge is held in place with screws that are between two and three inches long? Consider replacing

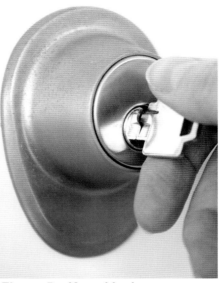

Figure 5 – Keyed lock

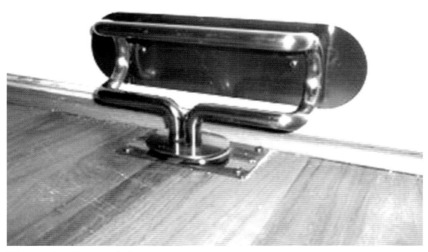

Figure 6 – Door club

them with deck screws that are at least four inches long so they will screw through the decorative trim and into the frame around the door, lending additional stability to your door.

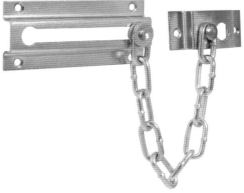

Figure 7 – Door chain

What doesn't work well?

Security Chains: Do you know the little chain on the door? Most of us have them. They usually come in brass, look nice, and give us a sense of security opening the door a little to speak to whomever is on the other side. I have one on my front door. I installed it before I knew better. If you look closely, the screws that attach the plates to the door and the frame are about one-half inch long. That isn't very long and it takes very little force to push the door open, stripping the screws out of the wood.

Doggie Doors: Surprisingly, many burglars gain access to a home by crawling in through the dog door. Before installing this convenience think about where it is. Does it open to the main home or to a mudroom that has another door you can secure? Is there a way to lock it closed from the inside so that it is not accessible to anyone on the outside? Some dog doors have a panel that locks into place on the inside of the door that prevents access. If your medium or large dog can fit through the opening, so can a small to medium sized person.

Alarm Systems

Alarm systems can be complex. Therefore, having them professionally installed and monitored may be chosen. You can also choose to apply contacts that make noise when they are disturbed. Some counties require you to register your alarm system, so check your local laws. The noise factor can be a deterrent, besides letting you know someone is trying to come in, but it could scare off the criminal (for some reason they seem to prefer not to attract attention to themselves).

The most simplistic device is a door wedge, very much like the rubber stoppers we use to prop doors open, except when you put this in place and turn it on it makes a lot of noise if someone tries to open the door. Their portability make them ideal for apartments, college dorms, even hotel rooms! They are also easy to remove if you have to get out fast.

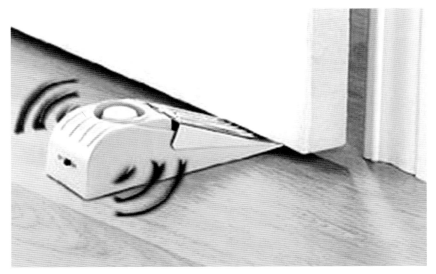

Figure 8 – Door wedge alarm

Exterior Landscaping

Be aware of what you can see as you are walking up to your home. Are there lovely full arborvitae near the front door? These can shield someone who is waiting for you, or block other's view of

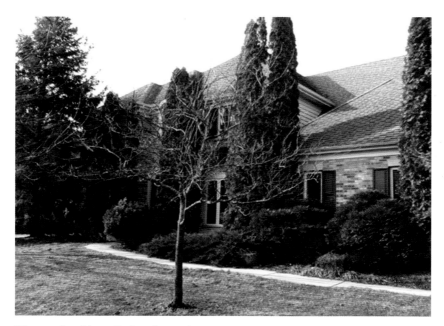

Figure 9 – Unsafe landscaping

the home if someone is trying to break in. Do you have tall shrubs near ground level windows? These also provide a place to hide, or a place for a criminal to work on gaining access to your home without being seen.

Don't let your landscaping obstruct your home, or your safety. Trees and shrubs can be lovely, as well as functional, just keep them pruned so they don't obscure the view. Consider planting thorny or pricker shrubs under windows, such as holly or haw-thorn. They will discourage most intruders and look nice at the same time!

Exterior Lighting

Security lighting can be one of the most significant improvements you make to the outside of your home. Sensor lights come on when someone approaches. These lights can alert you and save energy. If you have an exterior light that is on a switch, consider installing a sensor adapter that screws into the socket and leaving the switch in the on position. Solar and low voltage lights make great walkway markers and are also bright enough to illuminate an entryway.

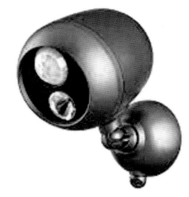

Figure 10 – Battery sensor light

Battery powered sensor lights make great additions to the rear of your home, such as on a deck or near a back gate. They will come on if someone passes near, lighting the intruder and giving you some notice.

You can also get motion activated sensors that beep inside the home if someone walks past them. They can be placed by your driveway, back gate, garage, or sidewalk.

In addition to lighting, security cameras can be a very effective deterrent. Don't have the money for a complicated system? That's okay, it is nearly impossible to tell real from faux. These fakes look like the real thing, are easy to install, and many use batteries to make a small red light flash giving an even more realistic appearance.

If you are in an apartment or rental property, consider leaving a large dog dish and heavy chain leash in plain view. Leave a pair of muddied size twelve men's boots you picked up at a thrift store by the door. Have a

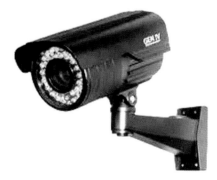

Figure 11 – Battery operated faux security cameras

friend's dog chew up a big bone and then set it out. Just move these things around periodically so they aren't always in the same place.

Garages

Do you have an electric garage door opener? Does it have a line hanging down with a plastic handle? Consider cutting off the handle, but leave the cord. This prevents a thief from using something, such as a long wire bent into a hook, to snag the handle from an outside window and open the garage door.

The door from the garage to the home should be as sturdy as your front door but often it is more like an interior door, with a flimsy lock. Many people don't even bother to lock that door with the misconception that the garage door is locked so the house is secure. Replace or use the temporary methods above to provide better security for this door. It's a small price for the security of your family and your home.

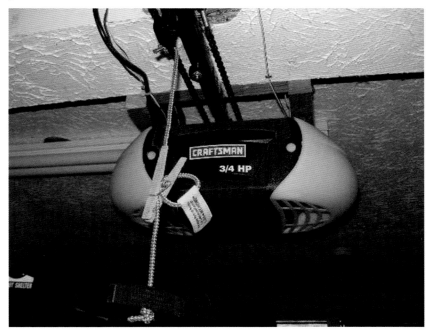

Figure 12 – Garage door opener

Backyard

Do you have a tall wooden fence around your backyard? If so, you probably have a gate. Most gates have one latch point, either at the top, where someone can reach over, or the middle where they can jiggle it loose. Consider adding simple latches at the top and bottom of the gate. Double protection against unwanted guests!

If you are in a townhome, condo, or apartment, consider how close the nearest neighbors deck or balcony is to yours. Can someone easily get from their deck to yours? If so, you can't count on them being as security conscious as you are and you need to ensure that windows and doors that are accessible from your deck or patio are secure. Being on the top floor doesn't make you invulnerable. If there is roof access, maybe via a skylight, someone can climb up and access your balcony via the roof. Unfortunately, I know someone this happened to, so it is a real possibility. Secure all exterior access to your home, just to be safe.

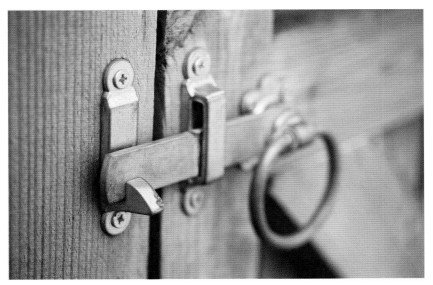

Figure 13 – Gate latch

CHAPTER 3

SOCIAL MEDIA AND CYBER-SECURITY

How fun are Twitter, Facebook, Myspace, blogs? According to statistics reported in 2011, 55 percent of Facebook users were twenty-six years of age and older. It isn't just for kids anymore. More and more adults are using social media to keep in touch with family and friends, reconnect with long lost buddies, advertise their business, or just update their entire social circle with one entry! I confess, I have two Twitter accounts, four Facebook pages, a blog . . . okay, maybe I overshare, but I launched National Take Your Daughter to the Range Day on Facebook and in five months it went from a new idea to a nationwide event with over one thousand participants.

What are the keys to maintaining your security in a world of oversharing? There are several. Probably most important are your security settings. Each site is different, but you want your personal information to be, well . . . private! Use the security settings to ensure that no one can see your private information. Once it is out there, friends of friends, and creative trolls, can find your information and deduce a lot about you. It may be possible to link bits of information and photos together to determine where you live and when you might not be home. It may also be possible to track information that can lead to identify theft, such as where you were born, you mother's name, pet's names, spouse's name, etc. A provocative picture may catch the eye of someone that shouldn't be looking. Ensure your kids' security settings are strong and help them understand the risks of sending out too much information.

Texting, tweeting, and posting, IMHO, has spawned its own language, a version of shorthand. You, as a parent, need to be as fluent as your teens and tweens so that when they are ROFLMAO @POS so DNR, IRL @ 8, you know what it means! IMHO, in my humble opinion; ROFLMAO, rolling on floor laughing my a** off; POS, parent over shoulder; DNR, do not reply; IRL, in real life . . . (that is a big one, especially if you do not know who they are texting). You can search texting acronyms and find whole dictionaries online.

One thing about the Internet—what happens in cyberspace stays in cyberspace. You may delete something but that doesn't mean it is gone. Our cyber fingerprints can remain indefinitely out in the ether. I attended an industry convention in Las Vegas not long ago. The joke

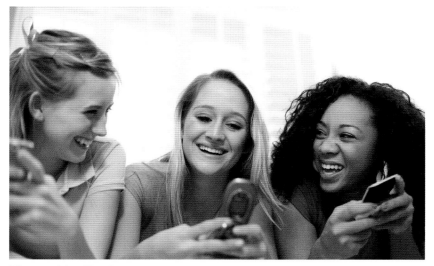

Figure 14 – Texting

among my friends was what happens in Vegas stays on Facebook! So true! I'm in photos of people I don't even know. Employers have been known to search social media to look for prospective employees. Think about how you want your persona to appear. Do you really want a potential new boss to see the drunken party girl, or would you rather they find a nice photo of you doing something with the family at the beach or a park?

Have you ever "Googled" yourself? It can be quite interesting to see how broad your presence is. Before I started writing and posting a lot, I was astonished at how much information I could find on myself. Currently, I can find several pages of references to me. Is that a good thing? Depends on the reference and who is looking!

Let's talk about the elephants in the chat room, the cyberstalker and the cyberbully. The cyberstalker can be just as scary as the stalker who shows up at your home or office, maybe more so because you don't know for sure what he or she looks like or who they are. It may start as a friendly "flirt" on a website or over email with just enough information to peak your curiosity. You respond and the chase is on. This may be a harmless flirtation OR it could escalate into something you aren't prepared to deal with. He, or she, may start slow to gain your trust and confidence, then slowly ramp up until the explicit nature of the contact makes you uncomfortable, but by then . . . he probably has more than enough information to embarrass you, or even find you IRL (in real life). One frightening aspect is what do you really know about this person? Only what they wrote to you, in other words, only what they wanted you to know and it may or may not be factual. Does he write things that give you a sense he has been to your home? Comments about where you were or what you were wearing recently? That would be scary enough but, he may escalate to threats, possibly explicit, excruciating detail about what he wants to do to you.

One truly frightening aspect of a cyberstalker is that it could be anyone! The boy who delivers your newspaper, the bank teller, the UPS driver, a coworker, or even a complete stranger! You can't go

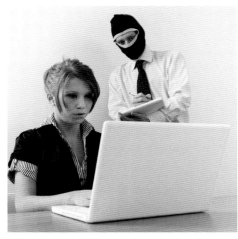

Figure 15 – Who is the stalker?

out without looking to see if someone is watching too closely, wondering; "Could this be him, or her? Is tonight the night they will try to hurt me?"

Being stalked is a pretty stressful experience but you can often figure out who is doing it. Cyber-stalking leaves you fewer clues to the identity of the threat. He, or she, doesn't have to reveal himself to you and you don't know who you are on the lookout for. If you feel you are being contacted inappropriately, save every contact and your response (if you respond, which I don't suggest). Take your file to the police. The laws haven't completely caught up with the technology but they are much better than even a few years ago. Being "targeted" is not a compliment, nor is it your fault. Waiting for the confrontation can be the worst part. If you have no idea who is targeting you, you can't watch out for someone, or you find yourself watching out for everyone! Keep records of contacts and suspicious behavior. Share these notes with the police, or at least with someone you trust. Stay calm but alert. If you don't respond there is a chance they will move on to a more entertaining victim. There is a chance that you can write a firm but polite go away, but if you do, don't respond to further contacts as this completely negates your initial rebuttal. If you do respond, it reinforces the delusion and may cause the person to escalate in their fantasy or delusion. You didn't ask for this, you do not owe this stranger a response.

Cyberbullying is becoming more prevalent, especially among teens. There have been instances of kids being targeted by peers, and sometimes even adults, with hatred and sometimes even mean, orchestrated campaigns of abuse. Extreme cases have ultimately resulted in suicide by the victim! Think about it, have you ever posted a snarky comment on someone's blog or a news feed because you could do it anonymously? Hiding behind a screen name gives some people the sense that they are not accountable for their words and they feel they can write things they would never say. If you doubt this, scan the comment thread on any controversial article on the web. They are likely filled with profanity, accusations against people who disagree with the writer's views, and sometimes even threats of violence. For many of these people, their "civility filter" is clearly OFF. It is that lack of consequences, or responsibility, that can lead some people to think it is okay to write whatever they want to. Sometimes this can incite others to follow along, topping each other in the escalation of rudeness and unacceptable vitriol . . . all while hiding behind their keyboard, knowing it is unlikely they will ever have to answer for their words. Or, at least that is what they think. Do not delete files if you find yourself under attack. Often the police can backtrack and find the identity of the bully. Even if a criminal charge cannot be brought, there may be a cause for civil action. Many schools have strong anti-bullying policies as well. Much like the bully on the playground that you can confront directly the cyberbully is usually a coward. They let their fingers do the talking, and scurry away if a light is shined on them or someone stands up to them directly.

What are your options? Consider ignoring it if you can. Report the incidents, file complaints with the school, the police . . . don't engage in response, that is what they want. Remember, bullies do not deserve your time or attention.

CHAPTER 4

CALLING THE POLICE

There are many reasons you might be calling the police. Some are emergencies and require dialing 911, others are less critical and may be better served by calling the local nonemergency number if there is one. No matter your reason for calling there are several bits of information you need to provide. In fact, having a cheat sheet near your phone can help if there is an emergency and you get flustered. You will either be in your home or away when you find yourself needing to call. Let's look in the home first.

Statistics, pesky things that they are, tell us most home invasions occur between 10:00 a.m. and 4:00 p.m. Really, most of us are at work, or home alone with kids. However, this doesn't rule out the shocking crash that wakes you from a sound sleep in the middle of the night, making your heart pound in your chest.

No matter the circumstances, it helps to know where to go, a "safe area," and what to say to the police when you call. Your safe area is where you can effectively barricade yourself and your family if trouble forces its way into your home. You may want to plan for day and nighttime scenarios, just in case. Consider the layout

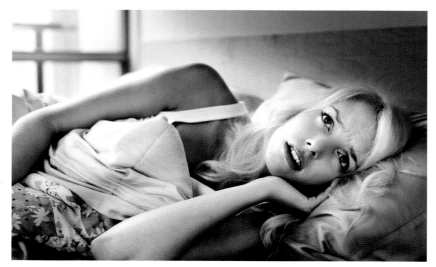

Figure 16 – Frightened awake by the crash in the night

of your home. Where are you likely to be? Where will the rest of the family be? What are the most likely entry points for a bad guy? From there you can figure out your best options for escape or barricade. If you opt to barricade together in a room you want to be sure that you have a phone, preferably a cell phone in case you lose your power or phone service, a window for emergency escape, and a sturdy lock on the door or some type of security bar to make it harder to force the door open.

Once you are in your safe area, or safe room, call the police. This is where the note card comes in handy. Think who, where, what, we, location, and information.

- Who—Provide your name
- Where—Your address and landmarks to find your home if you are in a rural or sparsely populated area, or what floor you are on in a multi-unit dwelling.
- What—Describe the circumstances, as in "Someone is kicking in my front door!"

- We—Describe yourself and who you are with (e.g., I'm a white female, five feet six inches, brown hair, wearing gray sweatpants and a white T-shirt, my husband and two daughters, ages seven and five, are with me).
- Location—Also describe where you are in the home (e.g., front left bedroom).
- Information—Let the operator know if you are armed, if you have pets, what, if anything you know about the intruder(s). Can you hear more than one voice or person moving through the house? If you hear voices, are they male or female? Give as much information as you can, from your safe place, about the intruder(s). Also, is there a way to get into your home without breaking down the front door? The intruder may have come in the back, but if the police pull up in front, that will be their preferred way in. Do you have a spare key attached to a bright heavy key ring you can toss out the window? Do you have a key hidden somewhere on your property that the police can use to get into your home? Key lock boxes,

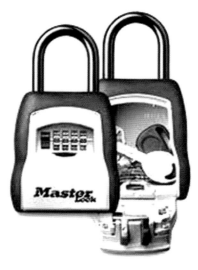

Figure 17 – Spare key lock box

similar to that used by realtors, are now available to the public and can be used to lock your spare key to a railing or fence. These have replaced the too easily found "key-rock,"or key under the flower pot, for many of us. Remember, the key-rock is a cliché for a reason, everyone knows about it, and that includes the bad guys!

Stay on the phone with the operator. He or she is your connection to the responding officers. If you hear a voice calling out "This is the police, you can come out," ask the operator for the names of the officers and then ask the voices on the other side of the door to identify themselves. Are the names matching up? If not, you know it is the criminal, and they can be pretty smart and tricky!

What about if you are away from home and something happens? Call 911 and be prepared to provide your name and phone number, location, and a description of what happened. Notice a pattern here? There is core information that you should have available whenever you call the police. If you dial 911 and are near a border (city, county, or state) be prepared to be transferred between emergency operators while they sort it out. This can be frustrating but hang in there. I was driving to work one morning on a National Park Service road. Just as I was taking the ramp on to the interstate, I saw that a car had flipped over in the ditch, the tires were still spinning so it was recent. I couldn't safely pull over so I dialed 911 to get them help. I got the county I had just entered and the operator informed me that was the adjacent county and transferred me. That operator informed me I was speaking with the Park Police and so they transferred me—by now nearly five minutes had passed. When I got to the correct operator and explained what had happened, they politely informed me they had already dispatched emergency responders. I was not the first to call. However, even if you think someone else called . . . place the call. Better to report the same accident three times than not at all!

Same principle applies if you are in an altercation or confrontation. Call the police! Imagine being in a mall parking lot and having

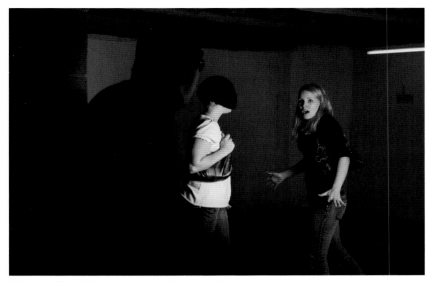

Figure 18 – Startled by a threatening approach

someone approach you in a manner you take as a threat and you yell at them to stay back and they run off. Call the police, describe the individual so they can be looking for him. The risk of not calling is that he goes around the corner, calls the police to report some crazy lady in the parking lot screaming in a threatening manner at him. Better they be looking for him than you! In the interim, he is mugging someone else! Rule of thumb, the first to call the police is the most likely to be believed.

Bottom line, if anything happens, call the police as soon as you are safe. Let them know so they can choose how to respond.

CHAPTER 5

DRIVING

TRAFFIC STOPS

No one likes to get pulled over. Sometimes it can seem like we're being singled out but if we're honest with ourselves we can usually guess the reason. Rolled through that stop sign? Pushed the speed limit? I was once pulled out of a pack of cars for speeding. In a Prius, going uphill. Did I mention in a pack of cars, all moving together, driving a Prius? Okay, we may not always know the reason why we are being pulled over, but we should still respond with care and respect.

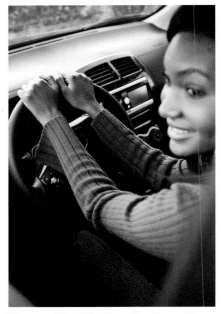

Figure 19 – Waiting for the officer during a traffic stop

If you get stopped there are a few basic guidelines to keep you, and the officer, safe and comfortable. First, pull as far off the road as possible. If there is nowhere to pull over, turn on your hazard lights, slow down, and head for the closest place to safely get off the road; this could be a side street, a parking lot, or a wide shoulder. Once you are pulled over, roll down the driver's window, turn off the ignition, and if it is low light, turn on your dome light so the inside of the car is illuminated. Then, place your hands together at the top of the steering wheel and wait. Keep facing forward; you can watch the officer in the rearview mirror if you want to. If you have passengers, instruct them to keep their hands clear and in sight, to remain quiet, and to face forward.

When the officer approaches, let him speak first, remain polite, and do not move or reach for anything. When he asks you for your driver's license tell him where it is and then slowly reach for it; "My license is in my purse which is on the floor on the passenger side, I need to reach for it." Slowly and deliberately get your bag, retrieve your license, etc.

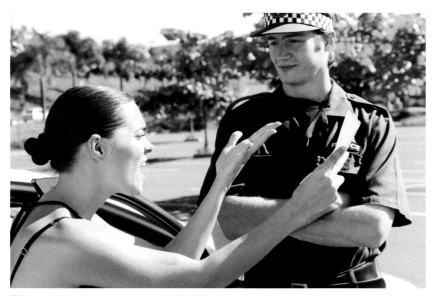

Figure 20 – Arguing with an officer is not a good idea

Whenever you are not responding to a specific instruction, place your hands back on the steering wheel.

No matter what, do not get angry or make any unexpected quick movements. A police officer is the LAST person you want to startle. Who knows, your good behavior could result in a reduced ticket or warning. But arguing will never help your situation.

What about an unmarked car? If you see flashing lights coming up behind you from a vehicle that doesn't look like a police car and you're in a fairly deserted area, what can you do? You may not feel safe pulling over where you are, and for good reason. This has been a ruse that criminals have used for years to entrap people, by impersonating a police officer, and pulling over innocent victims. Similar to a regular traffic stop, turn on your hazards and your interior light. If you can, drive at a moderate speed (but less than the speed limit) to a gas station, rest area, or other lit and populated area. Most officers will recognize that you are not trying to evade them, understand that you do not feel safe, and are heading to a secure place to pull over. En route, you can use your cell phone to call the police and ask if you are being pulled over by a legitimate officer. If not, stay on the phone while the police come to intercept the imposter behind you. When you do pull over, apologize and explain that you felt unsafe and were not certain that he was a legitimate officer so you wanted to go to a populated area. Why apologize if you don't think you did anything wrong? Courtesy! And, it helps to explain your fear so he knows you were not attempting to evade him. If you pulled over but the officer is not in uniform, you are within your rights to roll the window down and inch or two and politely request that he call for another officer. A badge, while a symbol of authority, may not be authentic. They can be purchased on line and at some gun shows. Criminals don't care that it is illegal to falsely represent themselves. If there is any doubt, request an additional officer or call the local police department for verification. Many states require police officers driving unmarked cars to be in uniform, but that is not a guarantee.

Breakdowns

That sudden unnerving silence from your engine as your car coasts to a stop. The *kaboom, ka-thunk, ka-thunk, ka-thunk* of a tire blowout. No matter what the issue, your first concern should be your safety. If you still have power, turn on your hazard lights and slowly make your way to the nearest safe pull off. If that means driving on the rim because the tire is shredded, so be it, your safety is more important. Get as far off the road as possible. Where are you? In the middle of a busy urban setting? You can call for roadside assistance. Are you in the middle of nowhere? You can still call, but leave the vehicle and get off the road and out of sight. Go somewhere where you can see your car but where you are not easy to see from the road. That way if someone pulls over they will see an abandoned vehicle, not a victim.

If it is a flat tire and you want to change it more power to you! Only change tires on the nontraffic side of the vehicle. You are too

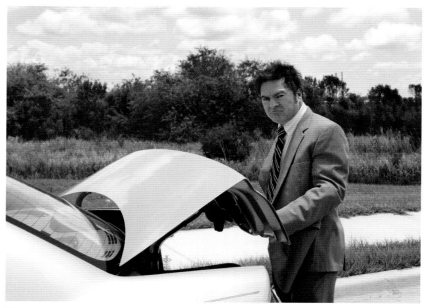

Figure 21 – Standing behind the car

exposed trying to change a tire on the traffic side, wait for roadside assistance. You've made the decision to tackle the problem, the spare is in the trunk, so . . . where do you stand? Behind the car? NO! It is easier, but you need to, as much as humanly possible, be beside the car, on the nontraffic side.

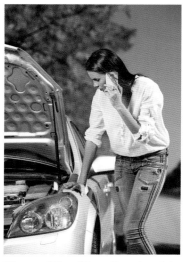

Why is it so important to be beside the car and not behind it? If someone becomes fixated on the flashing of your hazard lights and steers toward them, and according to emergency responders, it happens all the time, you do not want them to hit you where you are

Figure 22 – Standing beside the car

standing. At least if you are beside the car you have a chance. If you are behind it, and the car is rear-ended, you could be seriously injured or killed. This is also why police officers park at an angle behind another vehicle during traffic stops. If they are rear-ended, their car will move forward at an angle instead of straight into the car in front of them.

GPS System

The GPS, or Global Position System, is so common today that most of us have forgotten how to read maps! They come in our cars, on our cell phones, and in devices we can mount on the dashboard. When you hit HOME on your GPS, where does it take you? To your house? You probably have a garage door opener in your car (if you have a garage), maybe even a spare house key stashed in the glove box? If your car were stolen the thief now knows where you live and has a way to get in. My GPS "home" is set to the address of a shopping center a couple blocks from my house. Is your registration or an envelope with your address in your glove box? The thief who just stole your car knows that your home is probably empty and that you won't be home anytime soon. While we must have our registration, and usually insurance cards, you are safer keeping them in your wallet than in your car. There is no easy way to hide them so that a thief can't find them.

Fender Bumps

These minor traffic accidents, sometimes called fender benders, or bumper kisses, are not always what they seem; they can be easily staged and are a common ruse for thieves, rapists, and murderers. What is the first thing you do when someone taps your bumper? You get out to see if there is any damage. While you are looking over your car, you aren't paying attention to the driver of the car that hit you and you have now become a victim.

If no one is around, hopping out of your car and leaving yourself vulnerable is not a good option. Instead, turn on your hazard

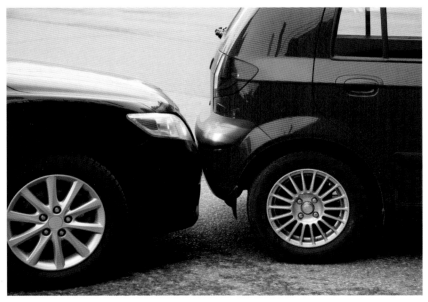

Figure 23 – Bumper kiss

lights, wave to the other driver, and make your way slowly to a safe area where you can call the police and exchange information. If your vehicle is not drivable, stay in your car and call the police for assistance. If you have no choice but to get out of the car, be very aware and cautious. Even the nicest appearing person can be a danger.

Carjacking

This is a scary fact: police reports tell us the majority of carjackings occur in parking lots and at intersections.

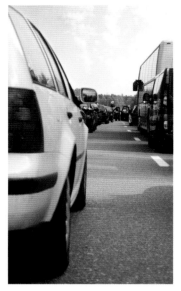

Figure 24 – Too close

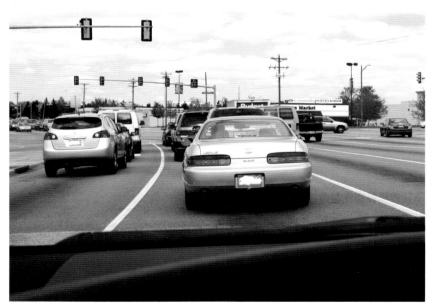

Figure 25 – Safe distance

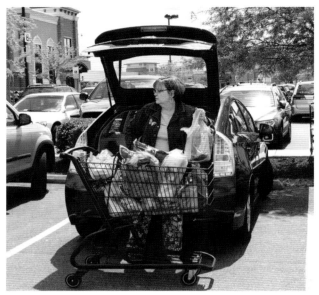

Figure 26 – Shopping cart as a barrier

What can you do to minimize your risk? First, keep all car doors locked. Leave yourself room to maneuver. If you can't see the rear tires and a little pavement between you and the car in front of you, you are too close. Don't let an irritated driver pressure you to roll forward, just because they want to be six inches closer to the light. This is your safety buffer.

If you are in a parking lot, there are ways to remain alert and safe. Are you loading packages, babies, or groceries into the car? Think of your "safety circle," a twenty-one foot radius around you (this is about two car lengths). No one gets inside your safety circle without you being aware and looking directly at them so they know, firstly, that you're aware of them, and secondly, that you've seen their face. If the person approaching you is thinking about doing you harm, this might make them change their mind and it gives you more time to respond. When possible, use your car's windows like mirrors to help see what is happening behind you. Trust your instincts. If something doesn't feel right, it isn't. Keep all car doors, except the one you are

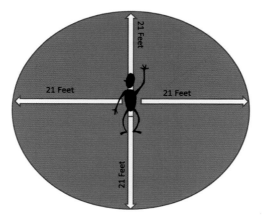

Figure 27 – Safety circle

using, locked. If you have a shopping cart, let it be a small barrier behind you. At least someone will have to move it to get to you, and you will have an extra second of warning.

CHAPTER 6

CAN YOU SPOT THE KILLER?

How often have you thought, "He looks like a nice person"? What is the most common comment made by neighbors when they are interviewed by the press after finding out the person next door was a serial killer? "He seemed so quiet, I never would have thought he was the killer" or something along that line. Truly, we want to think that we can judge a person just by looking at them, and we do it all the time. But how good are you at picking the right person at first glance? Take a look at the following photos and see if you can tell who is a killer and who isn't.

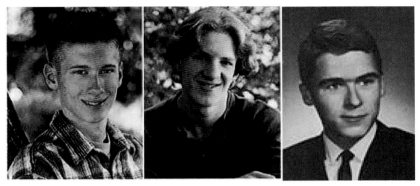

Photo 1   Photo 2   Photo 3

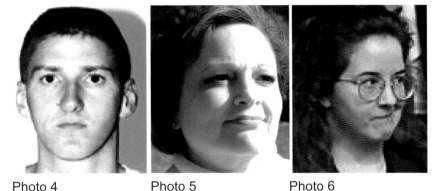

Photo 4   Photo 5   Photo 6

Figure 28 – Can you spot the face of a killer?

Can you tell? Let me give you a hint, photo 5 is your author, and no, I've never killed anyone. Look again, are you sure yet? It is impossible to look at a face and know whether this person is a killer and this one isn't, except in hindsight, when it is too late to save your life.

Photos 1 and 2 are Eric Harris and Dylan Klebold. They look like average high school students, but in fact on April 20, 1999, at Columbine High School in Littleton, Colorado, these two young men took fifteen lives, including their own.

How about the rest? Pretty average, normal, attractive even? Nothing maniacal or scary there?

Photo 3 looks like the kind of man I would have replied to on a dating site when I was single. Luckily, that never happened. This handsome charmer is Ted Bundy. He assaulted and murdered at least thirty women in the 1970s. He used his charm and good looks, often feigning an injury, to lure women to help him with seemingly harmless tasks, such as loading something into the car, where he then overpowered and abducted them. There may have been more, but he confessed to thirty killings before his execution in 1989.

Photo 4 looks like a kid just off the farm or fresh from the military. He is Timothy McVeigh, who, along with two other men, bombed the Alfred P. Murrah Federal Building in Oklahoma City, Oklahoma, on April 19, 1995, killing 168, 19 of them children, and injuring more than 400 people. He was executed in 2001.

Photo 6 is Susan Smith. This pretty lady was convicted of maternal filicide. She murdered her two sons, aged three years and fourteen months, on October 24, 1995, in South Carolina by strapping them into their car seats and sending the car into a lake. She claimed to be the victim of a carjacking and was shown on TV tearfully pleading for the lives of the children she herself had sent to their deaths. She is serving a life sentence.

In his book, *The Gift of Fear*, Gavin de Becker writes extensively about intuition and how you can recognize clues that you can use to save your life. Listening to your intuition is critical because, as you saw looking at these photos, you can't judge the merit of a person by their appearance.

The next time you look at someone and think "she looks okay," remember this chapter and judge them with more than your eyes.

CHAPTER 7

TIPS FOR TRAVELERS

Traveling—what is more fun than exploring some new place? Okay, not all travel is fun, and I admit traveling for business can be grueling. However, no matter why you are traveling, your safety should always be your number one priority.

First, plan your travels realistically. Trying to do too much, or waiting until the last moment and not allowing adequate travel time are not good ideas. As a result, these things make us rush, which can cause us to become careless, and that can put you in danger. Make arrangements with a trusted friend or neighbor to keep a daily eye on your home, picking up stray newspapers, packages, pizza flyers, and Chinese takeout menus. Have a neighbor park in your parking space one in a while. Use timers to turn lights on and off in different parts of the home, similar to the pattern you have when you are there. You do not want the house to appear to be empty.

Traveling is an art, and a balancing act. I used to travel a lot for work. Over time I learned to plan mix and match outfits and pack a few basic accessories. No one likes to drag large suitcases in their wake. These days my car is more loaded down when I'm teaching a class than when I'm going away for two weeks! The key, no matter your mode of transportation, is planning. Take only what you are pretty sure you will use, and leave room to bring home things you pick up along the way. I found myself in Dubai on business, and nearly had to buy another suitcase to get home (the market area was incredible!), but luckily, I was able to zip my bulging suitcase closed by sitting on it. And perhaps I'm even more lucky, it didn't burst open on the trip home.

If you are using any form of commercial transportation, at some point you are likely to hand over your luggage to the carrier. Minimize your exposure by using luggage tags that have a flap that covers your information. I write my name on one side of the little card, and my email and phone number on the reverse then insert it so only my name shows. If you were to casually flip open the tag you would only see my name. You actually have to remove the tag from the luggage to get it open. My tags are also big and bright and help make spotting my black suitcase easier.

When traveling by car I plan my route to take advantage of major roads and interstates, minimizing exposure to deserted highways and back roads. I also plan ahead to keep at least half a tank of gas in my car, which gives me an excuse to stop on a regular basis for a break. I try to avoid rest areas, preferring busier truck stops and restaurants near the roadway. These tend to have more people around, meaning there is less opportunity to be victimized. I also minimize my nighttime travel, preferring to get up at the crack of

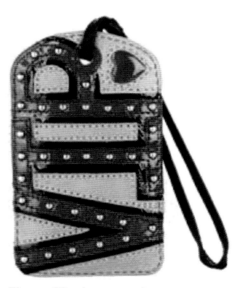

Figure 29 – Luggage tag

dawn to make the best use of the daylight. There are clichés about bad things happening in the dark, but the funny thing about clichés, they are usually based on fact.

No matter where I'm going, it's nice to know a little about the area before I get there. If you are going somewhere in the United States, you can do a simple Internet search and learn about local attractions, places to stay . . . dig a little deeper and you can find out about local crime trends so you have a sense of what to watch out for.

The US Department of State website offers lots of information for international travelers, including how to get help in a particular country, and travel advisories or safety warnings for specific regions. There are also many sites that offer specific information on customs, culture, and demographics for any country or area. These sites were invaluable to me as a woman traveling in the Middle East! I had enough sense to dress conservatively but wouldn't have known to hail a cab with my left hand, palm down (unlike the less studied tourists who were waving "hello style" at the cab that passed them by to pick me up further down the block). In my travels I have found a little courtesy goes a long way, and showing that you are trying to be respectful of other cultures can make your trip much more interactive and enjoyable. Another trick I learned traveling internationally is to always carry a business card of your hotel. When all else fails, you can hand it to the cab driver and he will know where to take you.

Even within the United States there are differences in cultures and customs. Depending where you are, if you want to order a Pepsi you ask for a pop, a cola, or a coke. Expect people to speak faster in parts of the Northeast, slower in the Southeast. Regional accents can sometimes be tricky as can regional idioms. Spend a little time doing your research and you will not only be safer, but you'll probably have a much better time.

One of the fun things about traveling can be your accommodations. These can range from a sleeping bag under the stars to a pullout sofa, or even a five-star hotel. I've tried them all. In my younger days I liked to camp in a tent, even though I slept with a hatchet under my pillow. These days, I prefer running water, indoor plumbing, and eight hundred thread count Egyptian cotton sheets. If you opt for a hotel or motel you can read reviews on most travel sites to get a sense of what others thought of the venue BEFORE you book your room. If you are staying in a high-rise, try to be between floors two and seven. Why? Ground floor rooms are more vulnerable to break ins. Rooms about the seventh floor are less accessible to modern firefighting and emergency equipment.

Once in your room, wherever it may be, look around. Check the windows, doors, balcony, connecting door. Is everything securely locked? Did you see a smoke detector? Sprinklers? Now, go back outside your door to the hall and note the location of the emergency exit. How many doors are between you and the exit? If it is dark or smoky, you may need to know how far you have to go by touch. Where is the next closest emergency exit? That may also be critical information for you in case your primary escape route is blocked.

In a fire, never open a door without checking to see if there is fire on the other side. How? Carefully feel the door with the *back* of your hand. Why? If you use the palm of your hand your reflex is to press forward as your hand detects the heat, risking a burn. Using the back of your hand will cause you to draw back from a heat source. If the door is cool, it may be safe to open, but if it is hot,you need to take other precautions to protect yourself. DO NOT open a door that is hot to the touch. You need to barricade instead. Soak bath towels in water in the shower or tub and use them around the edges of the door to seal it off. Call the front desk and let them know you are trapped in your room. If there is time you can call 911 as well, but start with letting the hotel know because their security staff will be coordinating with emergency responders. If you can open your window, open it just far enough to hang a pillow case out the window and close it on the edge of the fabric to hold it in place. The flapping pillow case will attract attention, while the closed window will minimize the risk of fire jumping to your room. If it is smoky in your room, you can wet a towel or sheet to cover your mouth and nose and stay near the floor to get the freshest air while you wait for help.

Most modern hotels use key cards with a magnetic strip on them, similar to Credit Cards. They are usually handed to you in an attractive mini pocket folder with the room number written on it by the check-in clerk. Once you get to your room, leave that folder behind. If you lose your key or forget your room number, the front desk can help you, just provide identification. But if you lose your key while it is in that folder, whoever finds it knows two things, your room number and that you aren't there. Be protective of your key card, they are easily erased; a magnet, such as on your wallet or purse or a cell phone can destroy the data on the magnetic strip. If your room happens to be some distance from the desk, it can be a long frustrating walk back to get the key recoded. As for the very popular Internet rumor that you need to take your key card home because if can provide all sorts of personal information to thieves, such as credit card numbers and address, this is myth and has been widely debunked.

Traveling can be a lot of fun, and safety doesn't have to interfere with that. Just be aware, do your homework, and enjoy your travels! As I was writing this chapter I discussed some of the tips with my daughter. Her initial reaction was, "Mom, you are just paranoid." However, she admitted that if we hadn't talked about it she wouldn't have thought of these things and that next time she stayed in a hotel she would be thinking about where the emergency exit was. There is a big difference between prepared and paranoid. Just because you're paranoid doesn't mean something bad won't happen, but being prepared can mean the difference between survival and disaster.

CHAPTER 8

OUT WITH FRIENDS

A very good friend recently shared a story with me about something that happened to her a few years ago. She was in her mid thirties at the time and was out for an evening with several girlfriends. I only mention her age to point out that

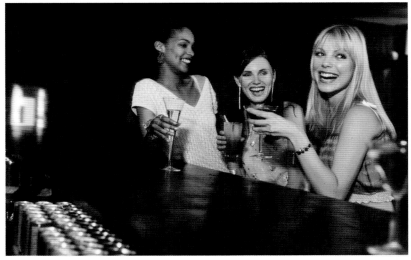

Figure 30 – A night out with friends

this isn't just a twenty-something risk. My friend, let's call her Nina, happens to be extremely chic and attractive, however, she is neither naive nor just out of her teens. This can happen to anyone, at any age.

At some point during the evening she began acting severely intoxicated, which was completely out of character and not in line with the little alcohol she had consumed. From that point on she needed to rely mostly on the accounts of others for what happened. She was said to be acting very "friendly with a man she didn't know," but also appeared to be very drunk, to the point of vomiting. Again, completely not normal behavior for Nina, but even if it were, it should have been a warning sign to her friends. Her now ex-friends thought she was having a good time and left her alone with the stranger despite her obvious impairment, that fact that she had consumed very little alcohol, and that this behavior was completely out of character. They later said they thought she was having a good time and was "into him."

For my friend, it turned out okay. The man, while a bit of a jerk, was not a "total tool" (Nina's words). He drove her home and

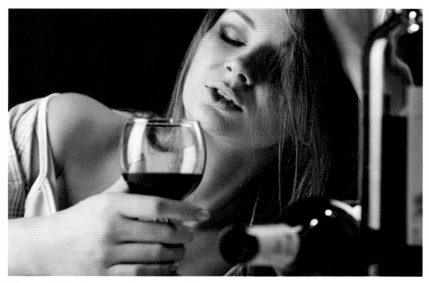

Figure 31 – Drugged or drunk?

accepted her resistance like a gentleman and left. She suspected another man of being the one who "drugged" her, and the two men were acquainted, which could account for him being responsible enough to see her home and not force unwanted attention. It could have been much worse. Again, her memory of that evening is very spotty, and most of the story was pieced together by asking others who were there, physical evidence, and the little that she did remember.

This can happen to anyone! No matter your age, looks, or how much you drink. Nina was, and is, a responsible adult woman who was out with other women she trusted.

Here are some ground rules to help protect yourself:

- **Never** leave your drink unattended, or if you do, and it wasn't watched, don't finish it.
- **Never** accept a drink from the hands of someone other than the server or bartender.
- You leave with who you came with, **never** leave your friend behind, especially if she seems to be impaired.

It is important to be reminded that danger comes in many forms, you need to be aware, and we all need to watch out for each other.

CHAPTER 9

CAMPUS SAFETY

Freedom! What an amazing time in your life. You survived the turmoil and torments of high school and now you're about to head off to college. You are young, free of parents (probably for the first time) and INDESTRUCTIBLE! Well, two out of three. As hard as it is to recognize, youth doesn't make you invincible. In fact, you may be more vulnerable because you are used to the watchful eye of a parent to help you be safe. The following are some basic tips to keep you safe while you are away at college, or even living on your own for the first time.

Whether you are living in a dorm, an apartment, a house off campus, or in a group environment such as a sorority or fraternity house, you need to remember some basic safety rules. Think SLAPP.

Situational Awareness
Locks
Alcohol
Pairs
Property

Situational Awareness is being cognizant of what is happening around you. When you are walking, or running, skip the earbuds so that you can hear people approaching. Put the cell phone away until you get somewhere safe and can text or call. Not long ago there was a video on YouTube of a woman walking through a mall and texting; she walked straight into a fountain. Funny? Oh yes! Dangerous? Very! Put the phone down and pay attention, not just at night but all the time. Walking and texting means you are not focused on what is happening around you. You could step into traffic, walk into a car, or you may not see an attacker coming at you. Awareness of your immediate surroundings, which I'm defining here as a twenty-one foot radius around you, or your safety circle, is a key component of your security. You don't have to walk around looking over your shoulder all the time, just keep your head up and casually scan your surroundings taking note of who and what is happening around you.

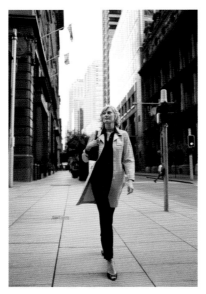

Figure 32 – Young woman walking with head up, alert

Locks should be a part of your day-to-day routine. Lock your windows, your door, car doors. Lock up your valuables: laptop, camera, cell phone, cash, credit cards, jewelry. All of these are easily transported, easily stolen, and easily sold.

Do you have a roommate or roommates? Ensure you are all on the same page about locking doors, controlling keys, and respecting each other's security. Even if you are making a quick dash down the hall or to the laundry room, lock your door. "Oh, it's okay, someone is in the room"

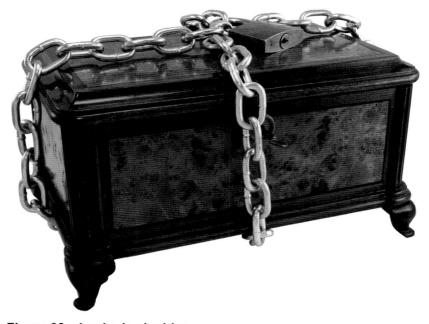

Figure 33 – Locked valuables

isn't a reason not to lock the door. If you are the one in the room alone, you may not realize that you have an intruder until it is too late.

Keys, if you don't live here, you don't get a key! Control the number of keys floating around! It is easy to give a key to your significant other so they can let themselves in, but what happens if there is a bad break up?

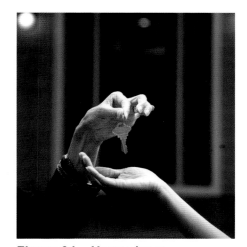

Figure 34 – House keys

Will you get your key back? Maybe! Better to follow the rule—keys are for residents ONLY!

Alcohol. PARTY!! Woo-Hoo! Okay, we all know alcohol is a part of college life for many students. However, the more you drink, the more your senses are dulled and the more vulnerable you become to danger. You already know this, but let me remind you again. Alcohol consumption slows your reflexes and dulls your cognitive ability making you an easy target. Does this mean I'm advocating for you not to drink? Legally you should be twenty-one to consume alcohol, and the rest is between you and your family. Out to a party with friends? Take turns being the designated "sober friend." One of you can abstain and keep track of the rest of the group, do the driving, and generally be responsible for the evening. Besides, someone needs to make coffee in the morning, and those that drank will be grateful for it! Take turns, trust me, the sober friend will have some stories the next day and isn't it nice to know someone will take care of you if you get sick?

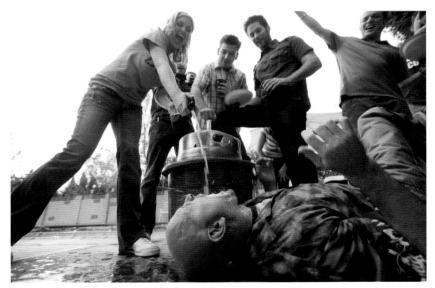

Figure 35 – Kegger!

The other serious concern with alcohol is binge consumption. The National Institute on Alcohol Abuse and Alcoholism defines binge drinking as a pattern of drinking that brings a person's blood alcohol concentration to 0.08 grams percent or above. This typically happens when men consume five or more drinks, and when women consume four or more drinks, in about two hours. First comes the buzz, then, if you're lucky, the vomiting before too much alcohol hits your bloodstream. There is a significant risk of alcohol poisoning, which can be fatal.

According to a Center for Disease Control report from October 2012, approximately 80,000 US deaths are attributed to excessive alcohol consumption each year, making it the third leading "lifestyle related" cause of death in the country. Additionally, under twenty-one drinkers accounted for 4,700 deaths and 189,000 emergency room visits for injuries or conditions directly related to alcohol consumption. These are very sobering statistics (pun intended). Be smart, have a sober friend, take it easy . . . trust me, you will have a lot more fun if you can remember it!

Pairs! Lots of things come in pairs: socks, dice, shoes. When you are out and about try to follow the "pair-plan." Safety in numbers may be a cliché, but it is also true. Walk with a buddy, take advantage of a campus security escort, let people you trust know where you are going and what time you are expected back. Minimize your solo time, especially at night. If you must be out alone, or even when you are with a friend, make sure you have pepper spray or some other legal means of defense. A flashlight shining into the eyes of an aggressor may temporarily destroy his night vision and give you a chance to run away. It is also good for lighting

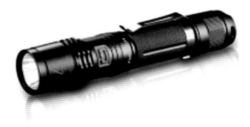

Figure 36 – 5.11 tactical style flashlight

up dark corners. The little flashlight you find everywhere isn't adequate; you need a bright light that has some "oomph" to it. Tactical style flashlights aren't cheap, but they fit your hand easily and are brighter than the key fob kind from the hardware store. Tactical flashlights can be found at tactical shops, gun shows, gun stores, and even on Amazon!

Property. It is yours, protect it! Don't leave your laptop or cell phone sitting on a table in the library while you go get another book. It may not be there when you get back. Hosting a party in your room? Lock up the computer, camera, cash, anything of value that can easily be taken. Being robbed is a very ugly feeling, especially when you know it was probably by someone you know. You can easily take steps to limit your risk. Gee, my closet doesn't lock, neither does my desk, what can I do? A footlocker can give you storage, and double as a coffee table! Plus, you can put a lock on it. Even a small luggage lock can keep out the light fingered party guest. A steamer trunk is another great option, it can be vintage or steampunk, covered in travel stickers or very simple. Instant secure storage. Yes, someone could steal your trunk, but people would probably notice. It is your stuff, it is up to you to protect it.

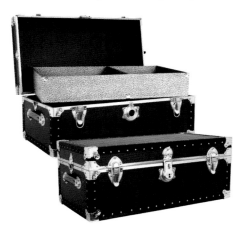

Figure 37 – Footlockers

CHAPTER 10

KEEPING THE KIDDOS SAFE

Keeping the little ones safe from harm is a goal of every parent, and it doesn't matter if they are three days, three years, or thirty years old, we want to protect them. The difference is how we do that. When they are infants, we watch them closely, screen our caregivers, buckle them into safety seats, childproof our homes—we do everything we can to ensure their safety.

As the children grow, and begin to assert their independence, heading off to school and playdates, we still want to protect them, but they are out of our sight more. As such, we need to teach them carefully how to protect themselves when they are away from us. One risk that our children face is being snatched: in a store, off the street, from a park. A moment of distraction is all it takes. You can minimize this risk by teaching children how to get attention when something is wrong. If someone they don't know tries to make them go with him or her, the child should yell, as loud as they can, "STRANGER!!" and keep yelling, "Stranger, you aren't my mom" or "You aren't my dad." Any adult in range will respond to the sound of a frightened child yelling "stranger."

Kids need to understand the difference between being polite and being safe. Unfortunately, the world can be a scary place. It is up to you, the parent, to decide if it is okay to respond to a compliment or question from a stranger if they are with you. What about when they are alone? Teach them they should keep a distance from people they don't know. If you become separated in a store, work out a plan in advance so they know who they should look for, such as a clerk or a security guard, if they can't find you. As long as you both know who they should go to, you will both be calmer, and you will reunite faster.

What if you need to send a friend to pick your child up from school or daycare? Do you have a secret code word for your family? Have you ensured that your child understands that this is a secret, only for them, and that it is how they will know that the adult who comes to pick them up at school was sent by their mom? Make it an easy word to remember that will have meaning for the family, but not too simple, such as the name of the family pet or the street you live on. Make sure they know that if the person who is picking them up does not know the code word, they DO NOT go with them. Many daycare centers require an authorized list of people who can pick up your child. You may need a code word for them as well, in case of an emergency.

These are not conversations you can have once and consider it finished. Not only do children need to be reminded of what is important for their safety, but the explanations and rules will evolve as they grow and develop and can process more complex information.

Teens are not exempt from safety considerations. One of the best agreements a parent can make with their teen is the commitment to have their parent get them wherever they are, at any time, when they feel unsafe, no questions asked. That last part is hard for many parents, but without establishing this trust the child may be afraid to call. As an example, your son or daughter is out with friends, the driver is drinking and your child recognizes the danger. Go get them. Maybe your daughter had a fight with her boyfriend and he kicked her out of the car, go get her. This agreement requires a high level of trust, on both sides, but it is critical that the teen feels safer calling home for help than going with the group. I've picked my daughter up in the middle of the night, standing on a corner, after a fight with friends. She was cold, crying, and scared. The last thing she needed from me was a lecture about staying out too late. She got a warm, safe ride home, some hot chocolate, and bed. The next day, when she was calmer, we were able to talk about what happened, but that was only because she trusted me to come get her when she really felt the need.

We would all do everything in our power to keep out children safe. The best gifts we can give them are security, confidence, and trust.

CHAPTER 11

SITUATIONAL AWARENESS

AWARE, CONFIDENT, AND SAFE!

As little girls many of us were given dolls to mother and told not to play with your brother's toy guns. Young ladies don't yell, they don't hit, they are quiet, demure—I even wore white gloves and a hat to Sunday school. Okay, I may be giving away my age here, but truly, girls are generally raised differently than boys. Most of us do not learn to fight, we learn to keep our discomfort hidden when someone invades our personal space or gets too friendly and gives us an odd feeling. This socialization, or conditioning, makes us ideal victims. We can be convinced that it isn't so bad, it is our fault for leading him on, we owe him, we are making too much of nothing, we need to keep our voices low. I lived the first thirty-plus years of my life like that. Shy, reserved, passive . . . then I woke up. It took a traumatic event for me, but hopefully not for you. I still behave like a lady, but only when I want to.

What does this have to do with socialization? Ever get that uneasy feeling when someone invades your personal space in the checkout line at a grocery store? It is okay to turn and politely tell them that you would appreciate if they take a step back. This is very reasonable, they do not have any need to see your pin number, or your transaction total, or anything else that is YOUR business. How often do we say something versus shifting uncomfortably and hoping they will get the message? What about the uneasy feeling you get when a stranger approaches you in a dark parking garage? Do you ignore that feeling or look at him directly and tell him politely but firmly to stay back? Some people are innocently clueless of personal space. More often, they are testing you to see if you will tolerate the invasion. For some, that is a thrill, for others it is a prelude to something much worse. Do not give them the "in." You can be polite in an initial encounter, but also be firm. Leave no doubts that you mean what you say. These are forms of aggression, or small attacks, and they can escalate.

I recently had to ask someone to leave a meeting for being a disruptive. I had already warned him several times, each time a little more forcefully. Finally, I stood up and told him he needed to leave since he was not able to control himself. He refused. I picked up my phone and dialed 911. He left, muttering profanities, but he left and did not return. I needed to escalate my warnings, and then back it up. I made eye contact, was polite but firm, and left no doubt that I meant it.

Sometimes you may wander into a situation without realizing it. If you are on someone else's territory, you may need to retreat. In those situations simply stating "excuse me, I am sorry for interrupting" and then backing away can be enough. In other cases, you can use your gender to your advantage and appeal for help, by saying I am so sorry. I am lost. Can you direct me to the nearest gas station, or interstate?" Trust your gut on this. It can work in the right circumstance, such as accidently wandering into a biker bar (nothing against bikers, some of them are awesome, kind, gentle people, but some groups can be aggressive to outsiders). Bottom line: get away from an uncomfortable situation fast.

You have the right to your space, your comfort, and your body. No one has the right to take that away from you. You can be feminine if that is what you want. You can be tough as nails.

Or you can be somewhere in between. What you do not have to accept is intimidation or aggressive behavior. Use your voice, stand up straight, make eye contact. No one can take your power from you without you giving it to him or her. You may have to dig deeply to find your inner strength, but it is there. Do whatever it takes to survive an encounter, be it eye contact, physically fighting back, or if you are mentally prepared and believe yourself to be in mortal danger, shooting your attacker. Remember, when someone attacks you, they have made the decision to do so. Your decision, your choice, is to accept it or fight back!

I have been told I project a "Don't mess with me!" attitude when I am walking. Some women are afraid that they appear less feminine that way, but I do not agree. I can project the same attitude in a skirt and four inch heels as I can in my tactical 5.11 pants and firearms instructor shirt. My husband actually finds it attractive. However, he also jokingly calls me his bodyguard. He knows I can take care of myself and that makes him more comfortable, but he also enjoys seeing me move with a sense of purpose and awareness. So, yes, I can be feminine and purposeful, even when I have to take smaller steps because my feet are killing me (but the shoes are so cute!). The attitude starts in your head; you decide that you are not going to volunteer for the role of victim. From there, you become more aware of how you stand, you automatically scan and become more aware of who is around you, and learn to make quick judgments of who might be a threat.

Along with your posture is "situational awareness," knowing what and who is around you. How do you know? Look around! Scan the area; are there tall shrubs that could hide an attacker? Is there a group of young men, or young women (girls can be just as dangerous, especially in groups)? Are they directly in your path? Maybe you should change direction. Do you walk through a parking lot with your head down, texting frantically like so many people we see these days? I actually had a young woman walk into the side of my car because she was texting and paying no attention to her surroundings. Are your arms full of packages and your purse dangling as you make your way to your car, only to realize your keys are in the bottom of your bag? You cannot stop every attack, but do not make yourself an easy target. Most stranger attackers will move on to someone who appears compliant and clueless if presented with someone who looks like they would resist, are aware of their surroundings, and will not be a compliant easy victim.

Above may be written from the viewpoint of a girl, but boys have similar issues. They may be more aggressive, but they still need to be aware, understand that their personal space is their space, be aware, and keep themselves safe.

There are many things to be aware of. If you are in a parking lot, do you scan the area, looking between cars, watching the area around you? Do you see someone looking at you and then looking at a third person and back at you? You might be a target. Get out of there or be ready to respond. Sometimes just the change in your demeanor, your posture, making eye contact can cause the bad guy to rethink the attack, but don't count on it. This is how they make their money, they can tell if your emotions match your physical response. Toughen up, and mean it. Remember, DON'T MESS WITH ME!

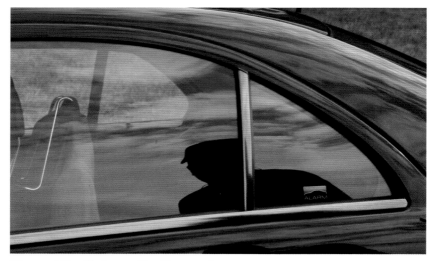

Figure 38 – Using reflective surfaces

Do you take advantage of reflective surfaces? You might see someone approaching by using the reflection in a car or store window. Do you face the ATM and stand close? Most ATMs now have mirrors on them, have you noticed that? Do you make eye contact with the person in line behind you at the ATM so they know you are aware of them? Attackers count on the element of surprise, they want to catch you off guard. If they know that you are aware of their presence and you are paying attention, they may very well wait for a more compliant, and clueless, victim.

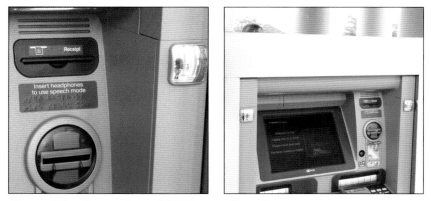

Figure 39 – Examples of ATM security mirrors

Remember, it is not just men, or people dressed in an intimidating style who can be a threat. Women and well-dressed men can also be a threat. Sometimes people work on a mixed-gender team. Ted Bundy found great success by pretending to be injured and in need of assistance to lure his victims. You can always say *no*! It is never rude to protect yourself. If their intent was bad, they may mutter expletives and move on. If they are sincere, they may be surprised, but that is okay. Reverse the situation. Would you rather someone deny your request for directions because they were uncomfortable or have them push down their fear and come to you? Still wondering? What if it were your sister, your daughter, or your best friend? You would want them to follow their instincts and protect themselves at the risk of being "rude" to a stranger. A common ploy is to ask someone the time. Simple, right? What do you do when someone asks you the time? Do you angle your wrist and look down to read your watch, thereby taking your focus off the stranger right in front of you? Or, do you bring your wrist up to where you can easily ready your watch and still keep focus on the stranger?

Lieutenant Colonel Jeff Cooper was a combat veteran marine and founder of the America Pistol Institute. One of his lasting contributions is the Cooper Color Code.

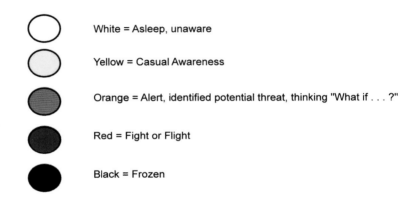

White = Asleep, unaware

Yellow = Casual Awareness

Orange = Alert, identified potential threat, thinking "What if . . . ?"

Red = Fight or Flight

Black = Frozen

Figure 40 – Situational awareness color code chart

Condition white is oblivious, asleep, completely unaware. Think of the person walking down the street, head down, texting away who steps off the curb and into traffic. They may be on the phone, listening to music, reading a book. What they share is a lack of situational awareness, and this makes them easy targets.

Yellow is aware, head up, confident, casually scanning your surroundings. You are not on high alert but you are aware of potential threats in your immediate area. It does not matter if you are ten or eighty years of age, projecting confidence in your walk and attitude can dramatically reduce your risk of an attack, or at the very least give you some warning that it is coming so you can prepare.

Condition Orange is when something catches your eye and something is not quite right. You may feel the hair on the back of your neck stand up, or an unsettled feeling in your stomach. Pay attention, something is off! It may be someone coming toward you. Flash mobs are a current danger, where a group of seemingly random people suddenly swarm together as a mob to wreak havoc. If you see people milling about and then they appear to catch each other's eyes and start to move together get out fast! You may see someone paying a little too much attention to you, and then glancing toward another person, they may be a team, targeting you. You may sense someone is following you while you are driving. You are in Condition Orange; you have noticed a potential threat. Now, start thinking "what if" scenarios. What will I do if he suddenly starts toward me? What will I do if that random group starts to move together? What will I do when I notice that car behind me has been there for a while? Even if nothing happens, practicing the "what if" helps you to begin to think about your response and keeping yourself safe. The more you practice "what if" the easier and faster the response becomes.

Condition Red is the Fight or Flight stage. The threat is there, you must take action. You can move from Yellow to Orange to Red very quickly, but as you become used to being aware you will recognize situations that have the potential to turn bad and will begin to give yourself more time to prepare. Later we will discuss various options for the fight or flight response, but the key is recognizing and taking action, thereby avoiding Condition Black.

Condition Black (which is not part of the original Cooper Color Code) is when you freeze. Time seems to stop, you cannot move, cannot think, and cannot respond. This happens to everyone at some point, but you must recognize it so you can shake it off and get back to response mode. Condition Black can be extremely dangerous, and very frightening. Just remember, it may feel like minutes but actually last only seconds, you need to push through so you can protect yourself.

CHAPTER 12

BASICS OF UNARMED PERSONAL DEFENSE

WHAT IS IN YOUR PERSONAL DEFENSE TOOL KIT?

What are the minimum things you should have in your tool kit? For me, the first is situational awareness. If you do not know what is happening around you, you cannot respond to it! Second, ensure that the "what ifs," that process of thinking what if "X" happens and how you will respond are present? I generally carry a flashlight, a Kubotan, pepper spray, a knife, a whistle, and a gun. I also have a voice and I am not afraid of telling someone to back off in a way that lets him or her know that to keep coming is NOT a good idea.

What is your minimum tool kit? Start with your brain! Situational awareness is the key to anticipating, avoiding, and responding to a threat. What should you carry with you?

Flashlight. You can find a small keychain size flashlight at a grocery store, a hardware store, or a large mass retailer. I once found myself in a parking garage at night during a power outage. I found my car with my flashlight without having to fumble in the dark. In a dark environment, a flashlight not only helps you to see

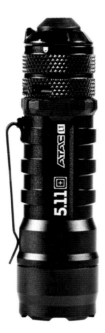

Figure 41 – Tactical flashlight

where you are going, it can shine light on someone who should not be there. You can also use a flashlight as a deterrent; you can flash the light in the eyes of someone who is a threat to you rendering them temporarily blind by destroying their night vision and giving yourself time to get away. There are tactical flashlights, about the length of an ink pen, but with a larger diameter. The on/off switch is at the rear of the flashlight along with a clip to make it easier to attach to a pocket. They may have a strobe function, and often a toothed bezel around the light to give you an extra impact if you have to hit someone with it by driving it into their face or hand.

Pepper Spray. This is a nonlethal option to deter an attack. If you get a keychain canister, do not get lazy and leave it in your purse while walking to your car. Have it in your hand or your pocket so you can get to it fast! Quick, get your keys! How long did that take? Three to five seconds would be pretty fast. An average person can close a twenty-one-foot gap in under three seconds. Can you recognize a threat, find your keys, and deploy your pepper spray in under three seconds? Do you know how your spray works? Have you practiced the activation and safeties? Do you know if it is a stream, mist, or foam? Do you know how to decontaminate yourself if you are accidently exposed? Sabre Red has the only formal civilian pepper spray training (Civilian Safety Awareness Program or CSAP) available as of this writing. If you cannot take a class, you should at least practice in an open area outside and away from people and pets and NOT on a windy day, to ensure that you know how your spray works and you have a sense of how to aim it to direct the spray into the eyes of your assailant. One caution, this is *nasty* stuff. When you are learning to use it, ensure that you point it away from your face and not toward an innocent person or pet. If you are accidently contaminated, flush the area with COLD water for at least twenty minutes. You will not be happy, but it is temporary. Many people think "I'll use wasp spray," or "I have bear spray for hiking, I can use that on an attacker." If you read the canister, it usually carries a warning along the lines of, "It is a violation of federal law to use this product in any manner other than described." So, as much as you may want to "sting like a bee" (thank you, Muhammed Ali) you should stick with pepper spray and leave the house and garden chemicals for the nonhuman pests.

Defensive Posture. When someone comes toward you, it is a natural reflex to square off to him or her, facing him or her. The hands come up in a protective gesture. Speak firmly and loudly, using as few words as possible. For example, "Get back," "Stop," "Go away," whatever words feel right to you. When I took the pepper spray class the first time, I called the instructor, who was playing the bad guy, "Dirt Bag." I was caught up in the moment; I actually like this person and felt bad later. Practice your commands until they are comfortable. Remember your social conditioning? We do not naturally bark instructions like a drill

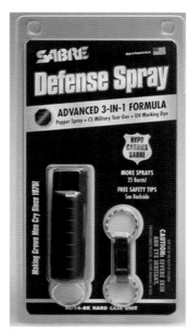

Figure 42 – Pepper spray

sergeant, but this is the image I want you to use. If they keep coming, draw your pepper spray and get ready. Keep your empty hand up to protect yourself and aim for the eyebrows so the spray will run into the eyes, even if he is wearing glasses. The effective range on most sprays is five to eight feet. A direct shot will temporarily blind your aggressor but his momentum may continue to carry him forward so you need to be somewhere else, to "get off the X" as my instructor likes to say. Move away from your current position, at an angle, as you are spraying so he cannot see where you are moving to. One final note on pepper spray, some states require that pepper spray be registered, or have a minimum age to carry it. Check your local laws before you purchase it to ensure that you are acting within the law.

Whistle. Another great item for personal protection is the simple whistle. Even if you panic and cannot get words out, if you can draw a breath, you can blow a whistle, making noise, attracting attention, and hopefully panicking your attacker. I keep one on my keychain.

Cell Phone. The last item in our basic tool kit is a cell phone. It does not do much during an immediate threat but can be a comfort right after. You can call for help if you are stuck somewhere, you can call the police, a friend, a taxi. Use yours to call the police immediately after an encounter. Tell them what happened, what you did, describe the aggressors, answer their questions . . . do not delay in making this call. The last thing you want is for the bad guy to call the police before you do and tell them there was a crazy lady in the parking lot yelling and making threats. You laugh, but it can take a lot of explaining if they track you down. In addition, the sooner you call the better chance there is of finding the creep before someone else is hurt.

What is in your hand already? Are you carrying coffee? You can throw it in his face. This should distract him, giving you a chance to get away. Keys, they hurt when you hit someone with them. Is it a mugging or robbery? Throw cash, or your purse, away from you and go in the opposite direction. I know the thought of giving up your bag or wallet is hard but everything in your purse can be replaced, you cannot. I carry my cash separate from my license and ATM card so I can throw my coin purse if I have to. If you can afford it, consider keeping a small stash of bills, maybe a lot of ones—sometimes called "mugger money," in an easily accessible place in your purse that you can grab and throw. Chances are good he is more interested in the money than in you. Also, make a list of everything in your wallet, or photocopy the cards and iden-tification you carry regularly,

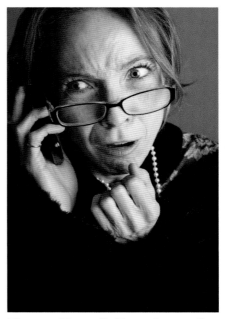

Figure 43 – Calling the police after an encounter

front and back, and store that in a safe and secure place, just in case.

What about other things you might have available to you? If you are injured and using a cane or crutches, you may look like an easy target. Take a few minutes to practice and get a feel for keep-ing your balance while using your cane or crutches to maintain distance from your attacker or to hit them. Thrusts can be effective and not adversely affect your balance. A cane can be used to punch or you can swing it like a bat. These techniques are best practiced, in slow motion, with great care to avoid additional injury. Anything you do to distract your assailant gives you a chance to get away.

Okay, those are the basics, but what about "weapons"? There are several great books that deal with an armed response and that is not the focus of this book, but here let us look at other options beyond the basic tool kit.

Stun Guns are effective. However, you must be close enough to be in physical contact, and you must maintain contact for three to five seconds for the effects to occur. That can be a really long time. It is not likely that your attacker will comply meekly while you are doing this. Also, while they make a very scary noise, a quick touch will not slow an attack (having accidently zapped myself with mine, I know, it hurts, but isn't incapacitating).

Tasers are also quite effective, however they take some skill to deploy effectively and since most are not easily "reloaded" it is not likely you will practice. In addition, the probes must be spaced apart, and penetrate the skin, so if there is a heavy coat, or one misses . . . well, it is not going to help much.

Knives take a lot of practice to use effectively. They are a close combat weapon, are not for the squeamish, and there is a real risk of having it taken away and used on you if you are not properly trained. Also, a folding knife may take time to deploy, open, and use. The best defense is a fixed blade used for thrusting. However, understand that anytime a knife if used, the odds are someone, probably both the attacker and the victim will be injured.

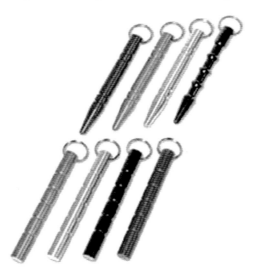

Kubotan use requires skill and training. It is essentially a stick, with or without a pointed end on it. There are many things you can do with it, but it does take specialized training. I do carry one with my keys on the end. It makes my keys easier to find, and I can always swing it.

Figure 44 – Kubotans

Physical Resistance

This is a big leap for most women. First, recognize that you are important; your life is worth defending! Second, remember, you did not start this. I have often said, "I won't ever start something, but I will certainly finish it." What does that mean? **Never give up!** If you are hurt, scared, feeling helpless—do not give up, keep resisting with every ounce of strength and resolve you have, you are stronger than you know, and you are worth it. Keep going until the threat is over; maybe you won, maybe he ran away, maybe you were able to run away, maybe someone came along and scared him away. General wisdom is **do not** go with him in the hope that you can get away later. It is more likely that your chances are better where you are then where you might be taken. Going to a secondary location usually ends very badly. It gives the bad guy isolation and all the power. Fighting where you start gives you the best chance of attracting attention and help or convincing the attacker that you are not an easy victim. Many of these attackers think of this as their job, and they don't want to risk injury that will either prevent them from doing their job or make them easier to identify.

Once he is no longer a threat you do have the obligation to stop your counterattack. If you continue once he is down, then you become the attacker and the law looks at you in a different way, so stop, escape to a safe place, and call the police.

Physical resistance is a learned skill. There are as many schools of thought as there are programs that teach it. Following is my personal philosophy. If you want to take formal training, I encourage you to search the Internet for "personal defense" training in your area. This is tailored more to street fighting, no rules, just surviving until you can get away. Martial arts are great exercise but many do not prepare you to defend yourself in a real-life situation. In addition, if like me, you are over forty and have your share of lingering aches and pains from pushing too hard in the younger years, martial arts can be daunting or impossible. I opted to take personalized one-on-one coaching in the Tony Blauer Spontaneous Protection Enabling Accelerated Response (SPEAR) program. I wanted to learn basic defensive techniques that I could do with my limitations, in the hope that I would never need them.

Women do not usually grow up learning to throw a punch. However, we can be very strong with an open hand. Try this exercise, have someone grab your arm and pull. What happened? Now, splay your fingers wide, tense your arm, and have the same person pull your arm. Notice a difference?

Your situational awareness should be on high alert when a potential threat is within striking distance. Watch them closely, they will telegraph their moves. For example, right before delivering a blow to the jaw, commonly called a "haymaker," you may hear an intake of breath, you may see a narrowing of the eyes, or a baring of

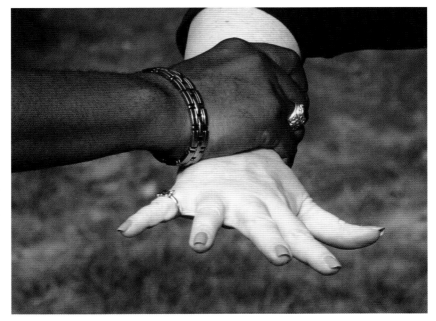

Figure 45 – Splayed fingers

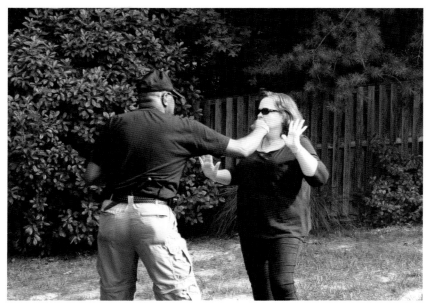

Figure 46 – Incoming haymaker

the teeth. You will see the body rotate away from you slightly as the arm draws back and the hand forms a fist.

This all happens very fast, but if you are alert to it, you will see it and the foreknowledge can give you an advantage. You have spotted the signals, be ready, if it connects, it will HURT! Let your head rotate with the punch, do not try to resist, that makes it worse, and you could be seriously injured. The key is to react to what you see coming to avoid the impact. Remember the extra strength you felt with the open hand? Now is the time to use that to your advantage as you raise your arms to deflect the blow. Then turn into him, rolling through, as you push him back and off-balance.

One of the most frightening scenarios is the grab from behind. If you are aware, you will sense someone approaching behind you. It could be a scrape of a shoe, it could be an intake of breath, a low growl sound, even a feeling in your gut, but you just know. This gives you a moment to start to respond. Raise your shoulders;

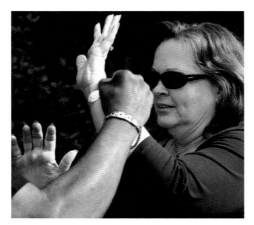

Figure 47 – Initial block

this protects your neck if you are grabbed around the throat. If you have time, bring your hands up so that if you are grabbed in a bear hug your hands are on the inside of the clutch.

Your focus is on getting him off you. The strongest places on a woman's body are the heel of her hand, the outside edge of her forearm, her elbow, and

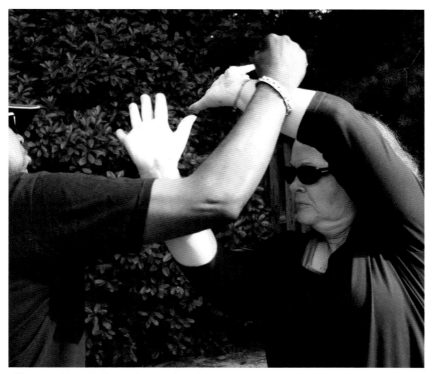

Figure 48 – Follow through with other arm to block

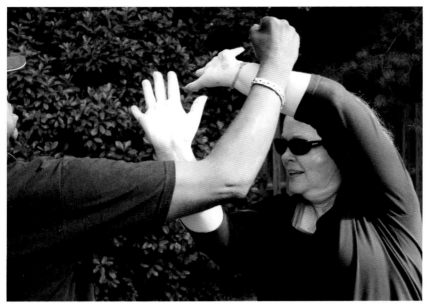

Figure 49 – Begin to push back

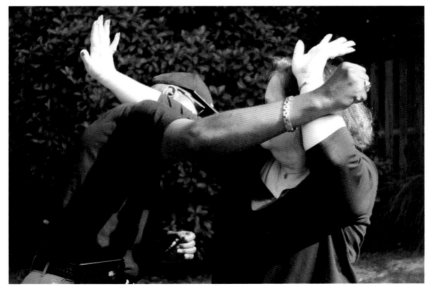

Figure 50 – Slide inside arm against the neck while keeping the fist away from your face

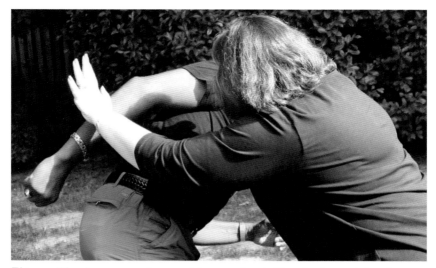

Figure 51 – Leverage by pushing and rotating to force him down

her knee. You can do a lot of damage and give yourself time to get away. One of your top priorities, besides yelling your head off, is

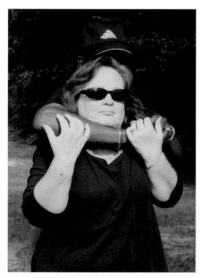

Figure 52 – Neck grab from behind (notice shoulders)

getting your hands free. Try standing a couple inches away from a wall; place your forearms, palms to elbows, flat on the wall, now lean in with your full body weight. Okay, push back. Not easy! You probably can't push him off you in that manner, either. Now, slide your arms straight up. It works! Same thing if you are trapped in a hold. You cannot push his arms away, but you can move yours up and free.

Once your arms are free, you have options. Rotate toward him. Remember, you probably can't push him off you, you need to go on the offensive. Reach for his face with an open, claw-like hand. Land just above the eyes and rake down. Yes, you may be a little squeamish, but remember, to your knowledge, you are fighting for your life. Stick your fingers in his eyes and pull downward. Show him the same mercy he is showing you, or is not showing you actually. Remember,

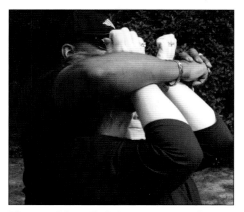

Figure 53 – Raising arms to break the grasp

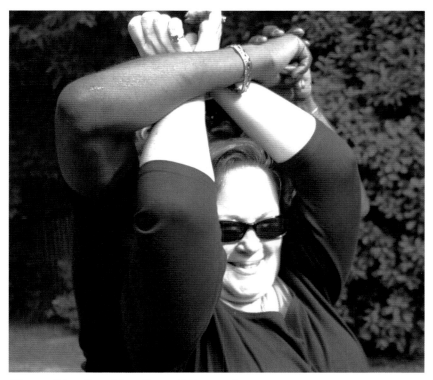

Figure 54 – Breaking free of the grab

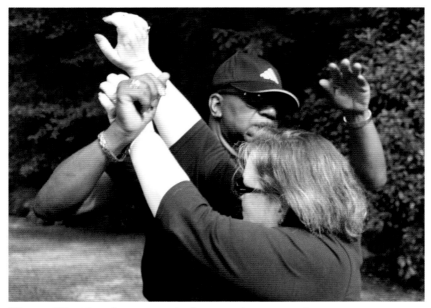

Figure 55 – Turning to push the attacker away from you

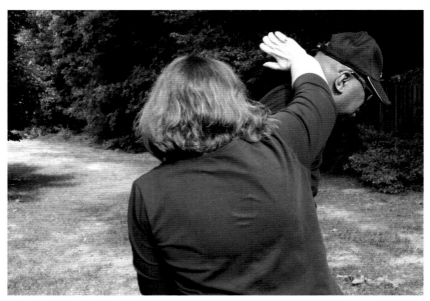

Figure 56 – Rotating through to put your attacker off-balance

he started it! Turn into him, pushing with the side of your forearm against the side of his neck to put him back and off-balance. Put your whole body into it, and really push while turning in toward him; this will help to drive him off-balance. You can thrust the heel of your hand under the jaw, causing his teeth to knock together and drive the head back. You want him to fall or be distracted so you have a chance to run. It does not matter if you are ninety-five pounds soaking wet, or two hundred pounds. You are stronger than you know.

You can also use your elbow to land a hit to the ribs or the jaw. Be aware of telegraphing your moves, which means giving him a clue of what you are about to do, such as drawing back for a hit, or being tentative in your initial strike, and keep your hands open with your fingers splayed to maximize your strength. Hitting with a closed fist is an easy way to break fingers and other small bones in your hand. You can land a hard blow, even without drawing back.

There are the classics that most of us know if you are grabbed from behind. If you can accurately judge where he is, you can try stomping on the top of his foot. Not great if you are wearing sneakers, but it works wonders if you are wearing a hard sole shoe or high heels! The other classic is the shin rake where you kick back and rake your shoe down the front of his shin; again this works best with a hard sole or heel.

Some recommend letting your body go slack, or "dead weight." The effectiveness of this will vary with size. Men

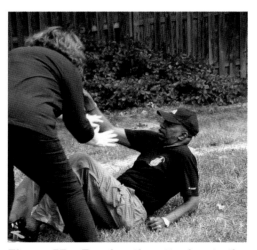

Figure 57 – Forcing the attacker to the ground

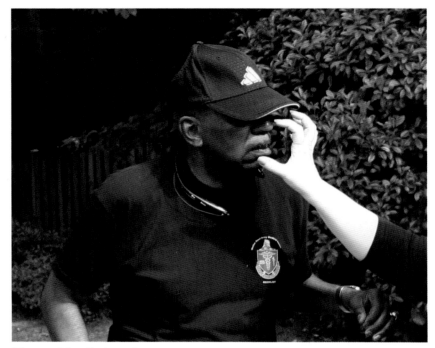

Figure 58 – Face rake

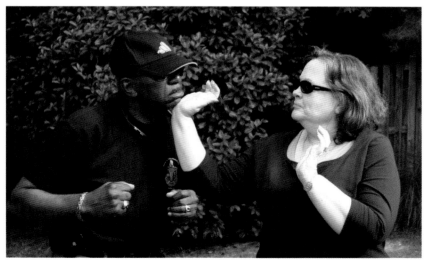

Figure 59 – Thrust to the chin

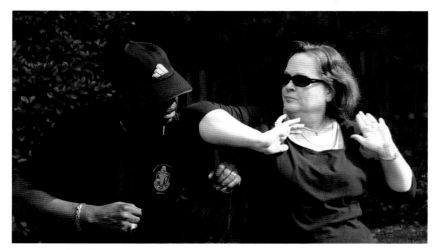

Figure 60 – Elbow to the jaw

tend to be stronger, so you could end up dangling by your neck and be in a lot more trouble than before. This is a judgment call based on your situation. In most cases, it is probably not a good idea.

But Lynne, what about the fancy kicks we have all seen on TV? Ah, if only it were true. Even if you have the flexibility of a Radio City Rockette and try to land a high kick, what do you do when he grabs your foot? Now what? You are on one foot, off-balance, and he is in control.

If you are knocked to the ground, remember to bring your arms and knees up to protect yourself, almost into a fetal position. Keep your hands up by your face, elbows out to block, knees up and ready to help protect

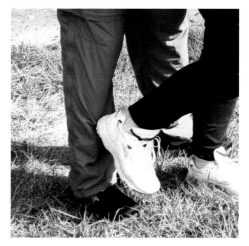

Figure 61 – Shin rake

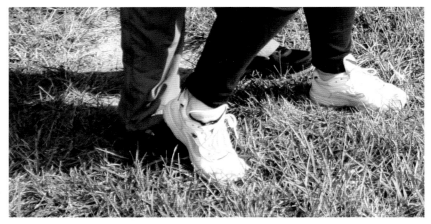

Figure 62 – Foot stomp

your more vulnerable midsection. You can twist your body to block an incoming blow and minimize the injury. If you get the chance to kick him, turn your foot sideways to maximize the surface area you are using to connect and minimize the risk of sliding off your target. You want to deliver a blow that will make him think twice about coming close. Sometimes, you just need to buy a few precious seconds before help comes along, or you have a chance to run.

If you are on your back, you may have a chance to deliver a sharp, and potentially disabling, kick to the groin. Do not be tentative . . . he is trying to hurt you. You may also be in a position to deliver a sharp kick to his shin, or knee, potentially knocking him off-balance and giving you a chance to get up and run. If you are kicking his leg turn your foot sideways to deliver the maximum impact and minimize the risk of deflecting off his leg.

Like everything else, practice, practice, practice. I have a heavy bag in my backyard. Not only do I wail on it to release stress, I practice hitting it, kicking it, pushing it, and raking it. I also have been known to try various combinations of hits: standing, lying on the ground, practing a hard strike, stepping back and then drawing my gun (either a blue gun trainer or having triple checked to ensure that it is unloaded). Practice helps me build my skills and gives me more confidence if I ever need to use them.

The keys to protecting yourself are remaining alert, not giving up, and remembering that you have the right to defend yourself against an attack. You did not ask for this, you do not deserve it, and you should keep fighting until you win. The best fight is still the one you don't have. All the practice and training can save your life, but the only absolute protection is avoiding the fight altogether.

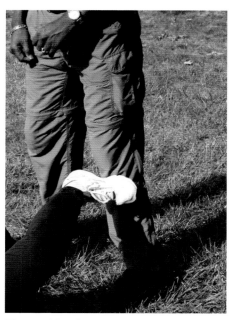

Figure 63 – Sideways kick to the shin

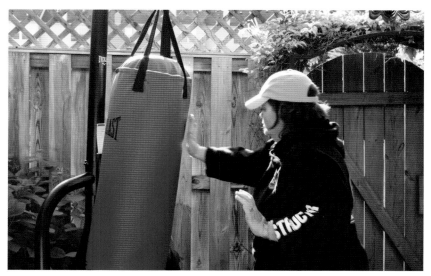

Figure 64 – Beating the bag

CHAPTER 13

STALKERS— TERROR IN YOUR OWN HOME

Most of us feel safe in our home, behind a locked door, with familiar and comfortable things around us. That changes if you have a stalker. You may not feel safe anywhere. Stalkers generally fall into two categories: a stranger

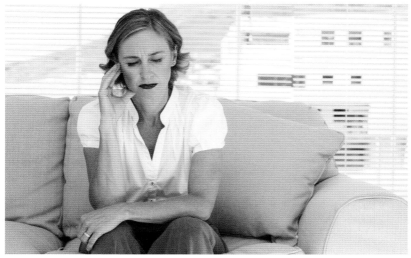

Figure 65 – Afraid in your home

or someone who is known to you, either casually or possibly from a more significant relationship that you ended. It is important to remember, you didn't ask for this, you didn't cause it. It is the stalker who is responsible. Second, don't feel like you are being paranoid, trust your instincts. If it feels wrong, it is! Stalkers come in both genders, and yours could be either.

Your responses are somewhat driven by the circumstances, but following are some suggestions. Don't stop here, if you feel that you are being stalked, or threatened in any way—call the police!

First, no means no. If someone is persistent, asking for a date or a get together, and you respond with a maybe or a yes to the third or fourth request, you have trained that person that persistence pays off. If you really aren't interested, say no, and then refuse further attempts at contact. This includes not calling to say thank you for the flowers that arrived at your office. No contact means no contact.

Keep a log. Record dates, times, and incidents. Keep a detailed record. If you have to go to the police or court, a record of the contacts or sightings will show the pattern of behavior.

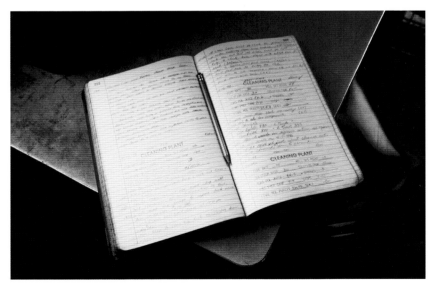

Figure 66 – Keep a log

Just because the creepy neighbor has been watching you from a distance and always seems to be there, doesn't mean he isn't dangerous. He just hasn't escalated. He may not, but you don't know. Don't take that chance. Many times an early intervention by the police can ward off an escalation, but nothing is certain. Keep your situational awareness, keep your log, follow your instincts, and seek advice from the police or a personal defense instructor.

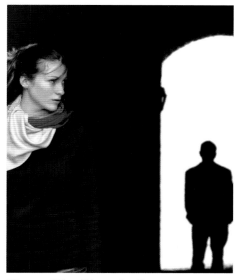

Figure 67 – Stay alert!

You are worthy of protection and deserve to feel safe in your home. Do not surrender that to a stalker without a fight.

CHAPTER 14

SAFE ROOM

A safe room is literally a place where you and your family can go in an emergency (the kind that doesn't immediately require evacuation outside, such as in a fire) and have some intermediate protection from the threat and access to tools to help you survive. Consider the likely entry points to your home for an intruder. Now, think about the composition of your family and if they can mobilize independently to the safe room if they need to be retrieved, such as a small child or an elderly parent. Next, think about the path from where you spend the most time in relation to the entrance points. Can you get to your safe room? Do you need more than one, sort of a "Plan B"? What about in the middle of the night? Can you round up everyone into one place quickly or are you on different levels? Does the room have one or more entrance points (more entrances mean more places to guard)? Is there a window to the outside (for escape or to throw keys to the police)? There are a lot of variables to consider when determining a safe room.

Once you have identified one or more rooms to use as a safe room (not a "Panic Room" ala Jodie Foster) you need to stock it.

At a minimum, have a hard wired phone, meaning one that plugs into a wall jack so it will probably still work in a power outage. Preferred is a charged cell phone if you get reception at your home so you can call the police even if your phone lines are cut. Refer back to Chapter 4 for tips on calling the police.

Other necessities are a good lock on the door or a brace to prevent it from being opened easily. A flashlight, in case you don't have power. Spare keys on a bright, heavy, keychain. If you are on an upper level of a multi-story home, no more than three floors up, an emergency escape ladder can be an option if you need it. If you are in an apartment or condo complex above the third floor, climbing out the window probably isn't an option. Do you have something to defend yourself with such as a bat or golf club?

If you have your family together in a room, where do you hide? Ninety degrees off the entrance to the room is your best option. Take a look at the diagram below and imagine your safe room. If someone comes through the door their scan will generally be straight ahead and

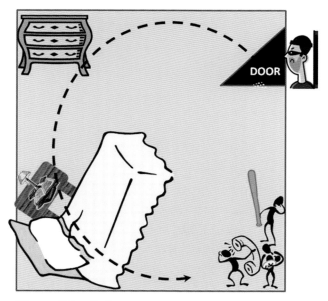

Figure 68 – Safe room

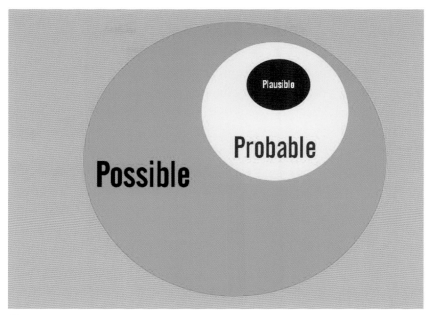

Figure 69 – Plausibility Principle

then around the room, ending at approximately ninety degrees. You want to be the last thing they see, giving yourself the most time to respond.

It is possible that you may have different plans to meet different threats. Consider the Plausibility Principle, this concept is borrowed from Rob Pincus's Combat Focus Shooting program, as shown above. Looking at the graphic where should you focus your attention?

The diagram helps you focus your attention. Is it possible? Sure, a bad guy might break in through your front window in the middle of the day. Is it probable? You live on a busy street and have holly bushes below your window, so the odds go down. Is it plausible? You have an unlocked window on the side of the house hidden from the street by trees and a fence, that is the more probable entry point. Thought of another way, everything that is plausible is probable, and everything that is probably is possible but not everything that is possible is plausible. So, where do you focus your planning? On the most likely, or "plausible" scenarios.

Think about your daily life, how many people are in your home, and the most likely entrances to your home by an intruder. Based on this information, you can make a plan for the plausible scenarios and decided the best evasion options for you and your family. It may mean leaving your home, or even splitting up. Whatever plan you choose, you should practice it with all members of your household and if you have regular guests, you should plan for them and make sure they know what to do in an emergency. The same way you would tell them where the key to the door is, they need to know where to go and how to respond if there is an intruder.

Plan smart, pratice regularly, and stay safe.

CHAPTER 15

HOME DEFENSE FIREARMS

You may decide you want a firearm for home defense, but which one? Several factors will play in your choice of gun, such as the configuration of your home. A defensive round fired from a pistol will penetrate multiple layers of drywall and quite possibly an exterior wall, and still keep going. This may not be a good choice for an apartment or an urban setting where all the homes are very close together unless you have clearly established your lines of fire or put up additional barriers to minimize the risk of over penetration. Plus, if you are going to keep a pistol for home defense, you need to practice with it. If you don't practice, you aren't likely to hit what you are aiming at, further increasing the odds of hitting something, or someone, you do not intend to. You have a very small tolerance for variance in a defensive situation, not all bad guys come in linebacker size. This ties back to one of the basic safety rules. Always know your target *and* what is beyond it.

Another option for home defense is a shotgun. Using defense rounds, which have multiple pellets contained in a shell, gives you a conical shaped discharge that allows for a better chance of impacting your target and reduces (but doesn't eliminate) the risk of penetrating walls. The shot will go through dry wall, but not usually as far as a pistol round. You still need to practice, but the tolerance for variance is much wider. I own a short pistol grip, 12-gauge shotgun for home defense. It is fired from the hip, not the shoulder, making it trickier to aim but easy to manage. The one disadvantage is most indoor ranges will not let you shoot one because it takes practice to judge what is level so you don't hit the ceiling. In the hands of an inexperienced shooter that can mean lots of damage.

If you choose a pistol for home defense, you have several decisions to make. Semi-automatic or revolver? Caliber? Size? Model? Based on medical studies it has been found that the wounding capacity of a .38 Special, a 9mm, a .40 caliber, and a .45 have only minimal differences. If this seems harsh, remember that we are talking about someone invading your home, while you are there, and threatening you and your family. The intruder may be armed, may be crazy or on drugs, or may just not care. You don't know. All you will know for certain, in the beginning, is that they do not belong in your home. I never encourage anyone to use a firearm unless there are no other options available to you. But, if you can't evade, and you believe that this is your only option, and you choose to use a firearm, you need to be competent and confident in your training and your practice, and then act with the resolve that comes from knowing you are using this as a last resort. Once the gun is out, be prepared to shoot. Thinking that showing a firearm will cause an intruder to flee has been proven false in the majority of home invasions.

So, revolver or semi-automatic? A revolver is simpler to operate, a semi-automatic holds more rounds. The trigger on a revolver averages eleven to thirteen pounds of pull, this is how much pressure you must exert with one finger to pull the trigger. Can you do it? Probably, with practice, but to be consistent you will need to build the strength in that finger. Conversely, the semi-automatic trigger pull varies, but is usually significantly less, often around five to six pounds. Why is this important? The faster you can pull the trigger, the more shots you can get on target. In the time it takes me to shoot five rounds from my .38 revolver, I can fire fifteen from my Glock 19 9mm semi-automatic.

Caliber? We've discussed wounding capacity, but what about the difference in recoil management? Recoil is the "kick" that results from the bullet exiting the gun. A higher caliber round will generate more recoil, and this can make a big difference in how fast you can get your sights back on the target and fire a second shot. Unfortunately, real life is rarely like the movies where the good guy only has to fire one round and the bad guy goes down. Videos of actual shootings show a wounded person continuing the aggression or running away, often for several minutes or longer before collapsing. Ask anyone who has been involved in a serious life threatening situation, such as a car accident or an assault, how long a couple minutes can be. It can literally feel like a lifetime.

So, if you want a pistol, perhaps because you can only have one firearm, and it will need to serve multiple purposes, I encourage you to look at a modern striker fired pistol, such as a Glock, Smith and Wesson M&P, or a Springfield XD. I recommend you look at a full sized pistol, or no smaller than a compact (such as a Glock 19). This will help you to absorb the recoil, thus increasing your speed and improving your accuracy.

Lastly, caliber. I recommend 9mm. Not a significant difference in wounding but a huge difference in recoil. I did a test, shooting side by side with a friend (a strong male friend), me with my 9mm and he with his .45, ten rounds. A third person gave us a "Go," we drove out, fired ten rounds into side by side targets. Guess who went empty first? We reloaded, switched guns, and tried it again. You guessed it. The 9mm was first both times, not by much but my hand was a little more sore after shooting the .45. Additionally, the 9mm is less expensive to practice with than the .45 because of the cost of ammunition.

Practice is Critical to Accuracy.
Accuracy is Critical to Survival.

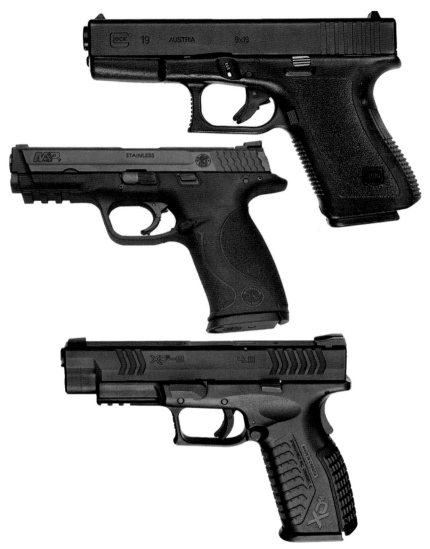

Figure 70 – Glock (top), Smith and Wesson M&P (middle), and Springfield XD (bottom)

You have made the decision to have a gun, you made your selection, got training, and are practicing. Now, storage? There are lots of options; many manufacturers make quick access safes that

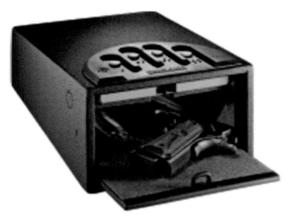

Figure 71 – GunVault gun safe

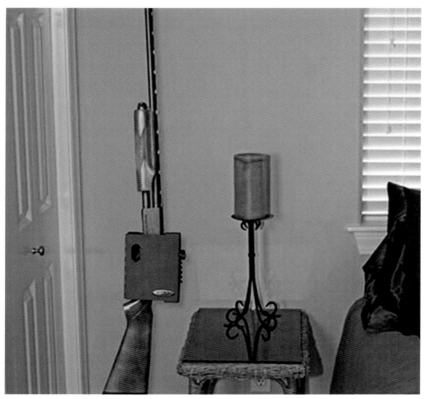

Figure 72 – Wall-mounted shotgun lock

can tuck under the bed, on the nightstand, or in a drawer. They will keep your gun secure, let you access it quickly, and many can be bolted to furniture or secured with a steel cable. Many people leave the safe in the master bedroom, which is also the safe room, and can simply open the safe at night for quicker access. It depends on your home situation. If you have small children who may wander into the bedroom in the night, you probably want to leave it locked.

The GunVault gun safe is great for keeping prying hands out while allowing you fast access when you need it. It has an eyes free keypad so you can open it in the dark, or when you need to keep your attention elsewhere.

Shotguns don't fit into nightstands, but that doesn't mean you can't secure one. You can get a wall-mounted bracket that incorporates a trigger cover, a quick release lock, and that secures to a wall stud. If you don't want it to be obvious, you can store it in a closet or behind draperies.

CLOSING COMMENTS

Whether you're in your home, out and about, or online—awareness and caution can minimize your risks. The world can be a crazy place. The only one who can protect you is you. It is smart to pay attention, to learn, and to follow the tips in this book.

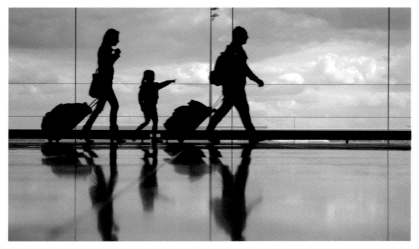

Figure 73 – Traveling with the family

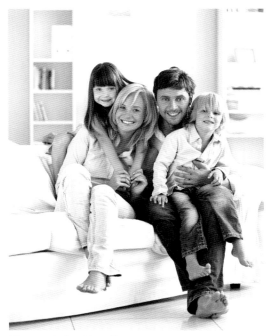

Figure 74 – Family

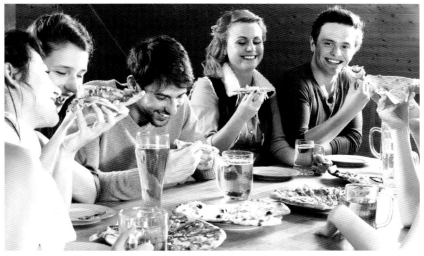

Figure 75 – Partying with friends

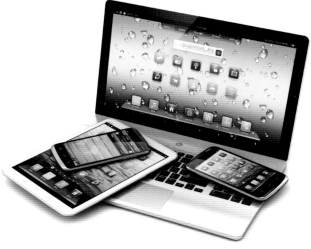

Figure 76 – Online life

Do things to make your home more secure. Plan with your family in case there is an intruder, know where to go, how to call the police. But before that happens do everything you can to ensure that your home is your castle, and as difficult to breach as possible.

If you are traveling, it is important to pay attention to the local customs. Being courteous to the local and their way of life will keep you safer during your visit. Traveling, at home and abroad, can be a lot of fun. Keep your eyes open, be polite, and enjoy your travels!

Be aware of your online profile and how open your life is to others. Manage your security settings, be careful about over sharing. Your friends know what is important, strangers don't need to know.

Watch out for your friends during a night out, at a party, at school. You have their back, they will have yours.

Anyone can learn to defend themselves. You do not have to be physically fit to protect yourself. Consider taking some basic personal defense training. There are many programs, but Physical Defense Readiness and Krav Maga are two of my favorites. There are programs for kids, teens, senior citizens, and there are caring

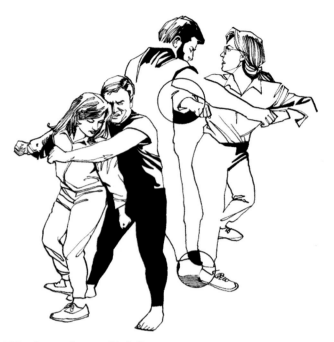

Figure 77 – Learning self-defense

coaches who will work with you and your limits to find a way that works for you.

Be strong, be aware, be safe!

ACKNOWLEDGMENTS

I would like to thank my family and friends for being supportive and patient while I bounced ideas off them and spent time at the computer writing. A special thank-you goes out to Becca, Tel, Becky Lou, Ben, Nichole, and most especially Mike Seeklander. Thank you Don for making such a realistic looking bad guy (he is really a sweetie). Thank you to the law enforcement officers who advised me on traffic stops and listened patiently, confirming my ideas. Thank you to Skyhorse Publishing, you all are awesome, but especially Kristin, the best editor in the world who offers not only corrections but encouragement!

Most importantly, thank you to the readers, without whom there wouldn't be a book! I wish you all safety and security in your lives.

ABOUT THE AUTHOR

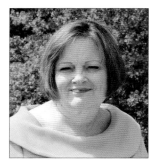

Lynne Finch is a firearm and personal defense instructor with Female and Armed. She holds NRA instructor credentials for Pistol, Personal Protection in the Home, Home Firearms Safety, and Refuse to be a Victim. She is also a Rage safety officer. She earned a Distinguished Expert in Pistol from the NRA/Winchester Marksmanship program in 2013. She holds a Defensive Firearms Coach credential from ICE Training. Her first book, *Taking Your First Shot* was published by Skyhorse Publishing in 2013. Also in 2013, she cofounded National Take Your Daughter to the Range Day, promoting gun safety education for girls of all ages. In 2014, the program was renamed Daughters on the Range because one day wasn't enough.

Her website is www.femaleandarmed.com. You can follow also her on twitter @FemaleandArmed.

YOUR HOME SECURITY PLAN

YOUR HOME SECURITY PLAN

YOUR HOME SECURITY PLAN

_____
_____
_____
_____
_____
_____
_____
_____
_____
_____
_____
_____
_____
_____
_____
_____
_____
_____
_____
_____
_____
_____
_____
_____
_____
_____
_____
_____
_____
_____
_____
_____
_____
_____
_____

YOUR HOME SECURITY PLAN

_____
_____
_____
_____
_____
_____
_____
_____
_____
_____
_____
_____
_____
_____
_____
_____
_____
_____
_____
_____
_____
_____
_____
_____
_____
_____
_____
_____
_____
_____
_____
_____
_____
_____
_____
_____
_____

YOUR HOME SECURITY PLAN

YOUR HOME SECURITY PLAN

YOUR HOME SECURITY PLAN

YOUR HOME SECURITY PLAN

YOUR HOME SECURITY PLAN

YOUR HOME SECURITY PLAN

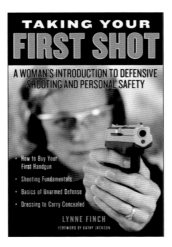

Taking Your First Shot

A Woman's Introduction to Defensive Shooting and Personal Safety

by Lynne Finch

Numbers don't lie; more and more women are purchasing guns and learning to shoot! While shooting used to be a male-dominated sport, women across the country have begun discovering that a trip to the range not only is relaxing, but also brings with it a sense of strength and empowerment. *Taking Your First Shot* is an introductory guide perfect for either those stepping out onto the range for the first time or those looking to brush up on their skills. Author Lynne Finch coaches women on the decision to learn to shoot, how to find formal training, selecting and purchasing a handgun, defensive versus practice ammunition, storing and caring for your gun, and concealed carry options.

Along with the shooting basics, Finch also teaches readers the importance of situational awareness and the basics of self-defense. Sometimes a gun isn't always an answer, and it's important to have a proportional response to the situation. Finch begins with teaching readers how to become aware of their surroundings, what to watch for, and how to respond.

$14.95 Paperback • ISBN 978-1-62087-717-3

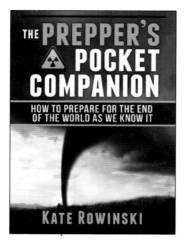

The Prepper's Pocket Companion
How to Prepare for the End of the World as We Know It

by Kate Rowinski

Most people don't believe they will ever have to face a real disaster, or are too scared to look ahead and quickly dismiss any thoughts of a future catastrophe. But a cataclysm can happen in an instant and without warning, and you won't be able to save yourself if you are not prepared.

The Prepper's Pocket Companion shows you what to do before, during, and after any disaster, whether big or small. With ten easy steps, you'll learn the basics of:

- Creating a foolproof plan
- Storing water and food
- Cooking off the grid
- Alternative energy sources
- Various disasters you may encounter
- Short-term and long-term self-sufficiency
- Safe and fast evacuation
- And much more

With this handy and instructive guide, you will learn how to protect yourself, your family, neighbors, and pets and be completely ready to face any disaster that may strike.

$14.95 Paperback • ISBN 978-1-62087-261-1

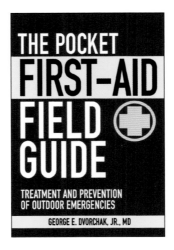

The Pocket First-Aid Field Guide

Treatment and Prevention of Outdoor Emergencies

by George E. Dvorchak

Practical advice for the on-the-go outdoorsman, this field-friendly guide is essential for anyone interested in first-aid preparation and care. Here is advice useful on a hike or for any fishing trip, including step-by-step instructions on dealing with fractures, suturing wounds, treating eyes and ears, managing allergic reactions, and more. With common sense advice, and in a handy, portable package, this is one little book that no one should be without in a campsite or in their forest hideaway.

$9.95 Paperback • ISBN 978-1-61608-115-7

ALSO AVAILABLE

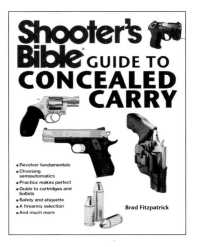

Shooter's Bible Guide to Concealed Carry
by Brad Fitzpatrick

Don't wait to be placed in a dangerous setting faced with an armed attacker. The *Shooter's Bible Guide to Concealed Carry* is an all-encompassing resource that not only offers vital gun terminology, but also suggests which gun is the right fit for you and how to efficiently use the device properly, be it in public or at home. Firearm expert Brad Fitzpatrick examines how to practice, how to correct mistakes, and how to safely challenge yourself when you have achieved basic skills. Included within is a comprehensive chart describing the various calibers for concealed carry, suitable instructions for maintaining it, and, most importantly, expert step-by-step instructions for shooting.

$19.95 Paperback • ISBN 978-1-62087-580-3

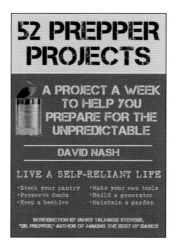

52 Prepper Projects

A Project a Week to Help You Prepare for the Unpredictable

by David Nash

Introduction by James Talmage Stevens ("Dr. Prepper")

Are you and your family self-reliant? Will you be able to provide for them and keep them safe? The best way to prepare for the future is not through fancy tools and gadgets—it's experience and knowledge that will best equip you to handle the unexpected.

Everyone begins somewhere, especially with disaster preparedness. In *52 Prepper Projects*, you'll find a project for every week of the year, designed to start you off with the foundations of disaster preparedness and taking you through a variety of projects that will increase your knowledge in self-reliance and help you acquire the actual know-how to prepare for anything.

Self-reliance isn't about building a bunker and waiting for the end of the world. It's about understanding the necessities in life and gaining the knowledge and skill sets that will make you better prepared for whatever life throws your way. *52 Prepper Projects* is the ultimate instructional guide to preparedness, and a must-have book for those with their eye on the future.

$16.95 Paperback • ISBN 978-1-61608-849-1

ALSO AVAILABLE

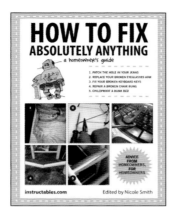

How to Fix Absolutely Anything

A Homeowner's Guide

by Instructables.com

Edited by Nicole Smith

There are a million things that can go wrong in your home. Faucets leak. Floorboards creak. Paint flakes. Chairs break. With *How to Fix Absolutely Anything*, you'll have step-by-step instructions to tackle even the most confounding repairs in your home, including:

- Installing a toilet
- Replacing the belts on your washer and dryer
- Patching up a hole in the wall
- Bringing a power adapter back to life
- Re-covering chairs
- Getting wax out of your carpet
- And many more!

From changing lightbulbs to fixing a kitchen cabinet hinge, *How to Fix Absolutely Anything* is a collection of the most indispensable advice and tips from people across the world who face the same problems you do. Hundreds of color photographs and easy-to-follow instructions make this book perfect for all levels of experience. It's a no-brainer for any homeowner, and the one gift to get any friend, family member, or loved one living on their own for the first time. Broke the microwave handle and don't know what to do? With *How to Fix Absolutely Anything*, the solution is only a few pages away.

$16.95 Paperback • ISBN 978-1-62914-186-2